To my parents, Dan and Kay Antonietti~
Thank you for giving me roots and wings.

Nurses on the Run

Why They Come,
Why They Stay

Edited by

Karen Buley, RN, BSN

First published by Dog Ear Publishing
4010 W. 86th Street, Ste H
Indianapolis, IN 46268
www.dogearpublishing.net

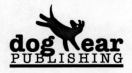

ISBN: 978-160844-336-9

This book is printed on acid-free paper.

Printed in the United States of America

Contents

Acknowledgements

Thank you to all who have been instrumental in the development of *Nurses on the Run*. Thanks to my parents, Dan and Kay Antonietti, who taught me to dream big. Thank you to my husband, Rich, and to our sons, Eric and Colin, for your support and encouragement as I pursued this dream.

Thanks to Terry Johnson, ARNP, RNC, MN who, at the 2005 Rocky Mountain Childbirth Conference inspired this book by asking the question, "*Who* will answer the call lights?"

Thank you to those who posted my call for submissions. Thanks to *American Nurse Today*, the Montana State University *Collegian*, the American Holistic Nurses Association (AHNA), the International Centre on Nurse Migration (ICNM), www.oklahomanurses.org, and www.nursefriendly.com. Thanks to Sandy Summers, RN, MSN, MPH and www.thetruthaboutnursing.org, and to Mandy Mayling, RN, HN-BC and www.brightestblessingscreations.com for publicizing my call for submissions with each deadline extension. Thank you, also, to the offices, clinics, hospices, and hospitals across the country who posted my submissions guidelines on your bulletin boards.

Thank you to my dear friends and writing colleagues. Thanks to Eileen Kennedy, whose keen eye and wise words were invaluable in the editing process, and to Kathleen Snow and Karin Knight for your suggestions and support. Thank you all for your friendship and for sharing my passion for this project.

Thank you to Eric Buley and Dan Warner for your assistance with my web design. Thanks to Mark Jackson and Amber Ortner at Dog Ear Publishing for answering my many questions. Thank you to photographers Agbeko Alorsey, Colin Buley, Rich Buley, Anna Knutson, and Eileen Moore for capturing our essence then and now.

Compiling stories for *Nurses on the Run* has been a labor of love. Special thanks to the nurses whose words fill these pages. Thank you for sharing your compassion, your humor, your skills, and your strength. It is because of your inspiration that I continue to practice the art of nursing.

Namaste

Introduction

At a 2005 childbirth conference the keynote speaker asked, "*Who* will answer the call lights?" The ensuing discussion about the ever-increasing nursing shortage planted the seed for *Nurses on the Run*.

My goal in compiling this book was four-fold: to inspire new and practicing nurses to remain active in their professions, to encourage others to become nurses, to offer suggestions to help remedy the nursing shortage, and to lessen the guilt of *my* planned 2008 exodus.

There would be stories—from nurses young and old, new and veteran, men and women, American-born and foreign-born, hospital-employed and community-employed; and information about the nursing shortage with words of hope for the future.

The seed flourished into more than I had envisioned, with an unexpected result. I would not accomplish my fourth goal. Because what I hadn't anticipated was that, prior to publication, the stories would inspire one nurse to continue her nursing career. *Me.*

Thrills, Guilt and Lessons Learned

Working night shift in OB, it wasn't unusual to field phone calls from worried parents about their newborns. Margaret, a recent graduate nurse, answered the phone in our Obstetrics Department early one morning.

"Hallo, we just have baby—" a male caller said.

When no question followed, Margaret asked, "How old is your baby?"

"One minute."

"*One minute?*"

"Ah, maybe two minute now," was the father's calm reply.

He told Margaret that mother and baby were fine, yet she advised him to call for an ambulance, and gave him the number. We prepared a room for mom and baby, and waited for our new patients.

After the ambulance brought mother and baby— umbilical cord neatly tied—to us, we nurses marveled at the stoic Laotian woman, and others like her, whom we had cared for during seemingly effortless labors.

Margaret and I reminisced about this as we manned the postpartum desk near the end of another night shift. Our co-worker Kim, working in labor and delivery, had called Dr. B.—the on-call doctor—for a laboring Laotian woman, pregnant with her second child. Margaret and I recalled the story from veteran nurse Sherry, who, noticing her Laotian patient was beginning to push, pulled back the covers and discovered that the baby's head was *out*. With Sherry's assistance, the woman gave birth—in her labor bed—to a healthy baby girl. It was remarkable to us how these women typically labored with quiet dignity, in direct contrast to many of our other patients.

When Dr. B. passed by the postpartum desk on his way to labor and delivery, Margaret said, "Let me deliver your patient! It'll be good experience—and you'll be right there." She motioned with her hands as she rehearsed emergency childbirth, "...and then you feel for the cord..."

Nurse-assisted deliveries were a rarity in our department. Protocol was in place: if the physician was absent and birth was imminent, we called for *any* OB or Family Practice doctor. If no doctor was present, we called for the Emergency Room physician. Yet, like with Sherry's patient, there were those unexpected occasions when babies came before a doctor arrived. On quiet nights such as this, we nurses talked through the mechanics of assisting with a birth, hoping that, *if* the unexpected occurred, all would go well.

Unable to persuade Dr. B. to let her deliver the patient's baby, Margaret retrieved the rolling ice chest and headed down the hall to fill water pitchers. I remained at the desk to answer call lights and the telephone.

Kim called for assistance to move her patient. "She's eight centimeters," she said, when I got to the labor room. After we transferred her patient from labor room to the delivery table and arranged her legs in stirrups, I prepared to prep her while Kim left to summon Dr. B. from the nearby doctors' lounge.

As the woman panted with rhythmic waves of contractions, I grabbed a pair of sterile gloves from the supply cabinet near the head of the delivery table. In my haste, I touched the outside of the second glove as I prepared to put it on. *Contaminated!* Not wanting to waste time, I staged a two-second internal debate, "Just put it on...NO!" It was only a small area that my hand had touched, I'd tried to rationalize, but if I used that glove, "sterile procedure" would've been a moot point.

I pulled off the first glove, snagged a new pair, and was quickly but carefully putting them on when I heard a guttural grunt behind me. Glancing over my shoulder, I saw in the mirror dark hair emerging from the patient's birth canal.

"KIM!" I hollered through my mask, as I hurried to the end of the delivery table. And to the patient, I said, "DO THIS!"—hoping to overcome our language barrier—as I blew hard and fast.

Instead, she continued to push. With one gloved hand, one bare hand, and adrenaline surging, I cradled her baby's head, and then body, as her newborn son made his way into the world.

Twenty-seven years have passed since I delivered that baby boy, but I'll never forget the thrill, the guilt, and the lessons learned.

Dr. B., bursting into the delivery room, calling, "DON'T DROP IT!" as, supporting the baby's head, chest and back, my bare hand slid down the slippery body to catch the legs. And later, at the postpartum desk, he asked why *I* had been in the delivery room, rather than Margaret. "*She* was the one who wanted to deliver that baby," he said.

Long before I'd heard about AIDS or had worried about hepatitis, I viewed gloves as protection solely for the patient. And that morning, *the patient* was who I was thinking of when I reached for the second pair. But had I known there wasn't time, that imperfect first pair would've served both of us better.

I learned that morning that haste can slow you down. I learned that hindsight is an excellent teacher. I learned that sometimes you are—or aren't—in the right place at the right time. And I learned that in nursing, as in life, being perfect isn't always possible. Being "good enough" may be the only choice.

Karen Buley, RN, BSN

The Nurse's High

It is exhilarating, and no amount of money can match that feeling.

That feeling of making a difference. You know, that indescribable emotion that swells within your throat, chest and gut and makes you feel lightheaded—as if you are high on something. That sense of well-being you experience when you are consciously aware that you have been a part—no matter how small—of something positive. Of something good.

During a twelve-hour shift, I transfused three units of blood to a patient who, when I came in, looked like a blank piece of paper. He was weak and slow—barely nodding or shaking his head to communicate. At the end of the night, just before leaving his room, I asked if the blood made him feel better. He said yes, and not only that, he said he felt alive.

When I said goodbye, he smiled. I was totally aware I didn't do anything major, but there was something about his smile. Although it was shy and faint, it was worth more than a million words. And it was more than enough. It was the kind of smile that made me believe that the minor things I had done actually counted.

I basically did the little things. I monitored him during the transfusion, made sure he was comfortable, and checked his IV site regularly to make sure the blood was transfusing smoothly and timely. I made sure he was aware of the possible reactions so he could get me any time he felt anything unusual. After giving him a diuretic in the middle of the night, I made sure his urinal was within reach and always emptied promptly. I made sure he had ice cold water because he always seemed thirsty. I told him I was there if he needed someone. I was there every time he needed something—the little, minor, unimportant things really.

I know, I did not write the transfusion order. I did not do the blood tests nor prepare the blood. I did not donate the blood. Don't get me wrong, I am not falsely and smugly claiming credit for all those big, major things. But still, it would be a lie if I said I didn't feel great, because I did. It felt great to be a tiny part of somebody feeling better. Feeling alive.

As if that's not enough, just before I left the unit, the charge nurse gave me one of those cards the patients fill out if they want to acknowledge the staff. Although the patient's name was familiar, I couldn't really put a face to his name. He wrote about feeling blessed that he had me as his nurse.

To be honest, it was a bit embarrassing that I couldn't remember a grateful patient, but at the same time, it was exhilarating. You know, that feeling that you made a difference, no matter how small, in someone else's life. That feeling, although incomprehensible, is just priceless. After all, at the end of a shift, when your back, arms, and legs are aching beyond verbal description, it is that something that matters most. The knowledge that somehow, in your own tiny, trivial, random, little ways, you made a difference.

That's all that matters. Everything else fades and pales in significance.

Lucy May J. Colegado, RN, BSN

From the Beginning

I began my study of professional nursing in 1958. What an opportunity to be educated in a baccalaureate course of study at Montana State University! I knew immediately that I wanted to be a maternity nurse since I loved caring for new mothers and their babies. It was a great privilege to impact families from the beginning. Nursing provided that niche for me.

After completing my undergraduate degree, I studied at the University of Pittsburgh where I specialized in maternity nursing. I became a nursing instructor, developed courses of study for prepared childbirth, and developed the role of the clinical specialist through my practice in a perinatal center.

A national study on perinatal outcomes in the United States demonstrated that we lagged far behind other developed countries in birth outcomes for mothers and babies. Multidisciplinary research to improve such outcomes allowed me to further enhance the practice of nurses via a program of outreach education.

Now it is expected that the care we pioneered in the mid 1970's—glucose screening—will be delivered to *all* pregnant women. This impact on improving health is only one of the ways that *you can make a difference* as a professional nurse.

An area of practice closest to my heart was the program I developed for families who had babies that were born with severe birth defects or were stillborn. The depth of sadness in these families is difficult to describe. As parents recalled their experiences, it was clear we were not helping them through the grief process. In fact, many had not even seen their babies after birth. This protection from reality was thought to be "helpful" and would ease their pain. Instead, it multiplied the disorientation associated with their loss.

Each family is unique and one story will grip your heart. I first met Katie, born in the late 70's, while her mother was recovering from a cesarean birth. Because of her complex genetic disease, we knew Katie's time on earth would be short. Katie's mother wanted most of all to hold her. Her father was very involved as well, and we began the planning process for them to take Katie home.

Parenting was a new role, and parenting a sick baby was filled with many fearful activities. Katie's parents were determined to learn about her tube feedings and everything necessary for her care.

It was winter, and we all hoped that Katie would live to see spring. We made arrangements with her pediatrician to come to the house when she was dying so that Katie would not get caught in the ER rush of resuscitation and subsequent life support issues. I was always as close as a phone call and made frequent home visits. The plans in place allowed Katie's parents to enjoy each moment with her.

Each day was a gift. Family gathered for Katie's baptism. She grew and gained weight and was able to go outside and feel the sunshine on her face. One May day the family went on a picnic. Katie took a turn for the worse and had great difficulty breathing. Later that day, she died at home, in her parents' arms as she "slipped the surly bonds of earth to touch the face of God."

Experiences like this are gifts that we nurses are given in our professional practices. I shall always know that I was honored to be Katie's nurse during her all too brief life.

I would not trade one day of my professional life. I will be forever grateful that I was able to teach those entering the profession and to guide them as they applied nursing science to patient care.

The opportunities are unending for anyone who desires to make an impact in the lives of people through the practice of professional nursing. Go for it!

Shirley Oscarson Wood, MNEd, CNS, RN

Shoebox Mysteries

It was time for spring cleaning and I was inside my closet, tippy-toed on a stepstool. As I reached for the last shoebox on the edge of the top shelf, my fingernails curled beneath the worn rim of the cardboard cover, edging the box closer towards me. Glancing up at the old box teetering above my head, I wondered what had possessed me to keep a pair of dress shoes for that long. Suddenly, the box gave way, contents tumbling onto the closet floor. Instead of an old pair of shoes, I looked down to see a familiar photograph floating to the ground—one I had stashed away during my first year of nursing. That photograph elicited powerful memories of an experience of awe and mystery from almost twenty years before, the kind of experience that keeps you in the profession of nursing, and reminds you of your purpose.

My first job as a Registered Nurse was in the intensive care setting, and I loved it! I signed up for Primary Nursing, which meant that I cared for the same patients every day until they went home, or until end-of-life. I was committed to Primary Nursing because it created continuity for patients and their families, and prevented things from slipping through the cracks in the large teaching hospital where I worked.

One day the Charge Nurse called me into her office, and told me that she thought I was too involved with one of my patients. She warned me about the dangers of losing objectivity, and recommended I take other assignments. I refused and left her office with an imperious stride. Later, I had to admit that she was right—I *had* committed the cardinal mistake. I had fallen in love with one of my patients.

My patient weighed two-and-a-half pounds. His mother was in jail when he was born, an admitted substance abuser and prostitute. His father was listed as "unknown." The day he was admitted to our large Neonatal Intensive Care Unit (NICU) his mom came to visit. I remember seeing the shackles on her ankles peeking out from beneath the hospital blanket someone had draped around her thin shoulders and lap. She didn't cry, or reach over to touch him, but she had the same sad look in her eyes that every other parent there had. She asked the guard to take her away, declaring his name as they whisked her off, "Demario."*

Demario had many problems: vision impairment, hearing loss, poor digestion, hip dysplasia, and brain scans revealing dark spaces. His prognosis for neurological improvement was poor. His worst problem was severe Bronchopulmonary Dysplasia (BPD) with bronchospasms, often requiring CPR when he became agitated. However, I knew him so well I could tell exactly what to do to bring him back: the right amount of pressure for the ambubag to open his lungs without causing harm, the correct head tilt to get his endotracheal tube in, and other nuances. I spent more of my waking hours with him than I did with my own children.

Reading his chart, most of my colleagues questioned why I even bothered with developmental stimulation. His chances for normal health and development were remote, but his other primary nurse and I wanted

*Name changed to protect patient confidentiality

to maximize his outcome, just as we would for any other patient. Our coworkers were glad that he had primary nurses, because as long as either one of us was there, they didn't have to take care of him. He was a "difficult patient." They shook their heads in disbelief as we continued to provide full support, but I felt honored to witness the glint of fighting spirit and desire to live that came through him, again and again. Something inside of me said to just keep on loving him while providing good technical care, because we really didn't know what would happen, and you never knew when an absent parent might come around, wanting everything done for her baby.

We kept him alive, and Demario grew. One day I looked at him and thought, *This is a growing baby, and his mom is missing all his 'firsts.'* I started taking pictures and made a photo album, including it as part of his Individualized Nursing Care Plan. Some nurses pooh-poohed these plans, saying they were just more paperwork. Anyone who took a few moments to actually read and follow Demario's plan, though, had a much better day when they provided his care. Over time, we weaned him off steroids and other medications. He became calmer, easier to care for, and some of my colleagues even admitted that he was "sort of cute."

One day I came into work after my weekend off, and Demario was *gone*. I stared in disbelief at the bedside where I'd worked every day for nine months. There, in place of his large metal crib draped with patchwork quilts, was a plastic isolette with a tiny newborn inside, being tended to by another nurse. Tearfully I glanced around the large room, hoping some kind soul had moved Demario to a quieter spot.

Instead, because the unit was full and Demario was a "Chronic BPDer," they'd tossed his belongings into a plastic washbasin and wheeled him away to the pediatric pulmonary unit, five floors up.

I was given another patient assignment that day and life in the NICU continued business as usual, though my heart felt raw, heavy, and full of grief and loss. The clinician in me knew that this is what we had been working for, to transfer Demario out of that noisy, invasive place. I hoped that someone would sign up to be his Primary Nurse—but no one did.

For awhile I visited Demario before going in to work the nightshift. There he was, sitting in his crib alone, beside himself, not knowing how to put himself to sleep. You couldn't hear him crying because of his trach. I would scoop him up for a quick hug, place him on his side snuggled into his favorite bear, and massage his head as he quickly fell asleep—the same bedtime ritual that I'd written in his Care Plan and that we'd shared for nine months. I stopped visiting after awhile though. His basic needs were being met, and I needed to let go. A few years later, when I worked in the Neonatal Follow-Up clinic, I looked for Demario's records. He was "lost to the system."

Eventually, I traded in the demands of intensive care nursing and the clinic to become a consultant for a medical products company. One day I went to provide in-services to nurses in a large hospital, hours away. To my surprise, the woman at the desk dropped her jaw as I approached.

"Karen Cooper, the nurse from The Children's Hospital?" she asked, her tone animated.

"Er, well, yes—"

She interrupted, "Do you remember Demario Johnson?"

I was stunned and embarrassed. For the life of me I could not remember who she was. "Well, yes, of course, I was his primary nurse in the NICU."

"Well, you don't me, but I know you. You don't know how many times I wished I could've met you! I saw your nametag—you see, I was Demario's foster mother."

Her eyes softened as she continued, "Years ago, I got a call from a social worker at The Children's Hospital, asking me to come and meet a medically fragile baby. Well! When I got there and saw that he was fifteen months old, had never been out of the hospital, and had a whole host of issues, I said no. I didn't want to deal with all the medical problems of a child like that, especially when there was no chance of reconciliation with his parents. However, that social worker knew me well and simply said, 'Just go and meet him.'"

"I went into his room, and noticed a plastic washbasin sitting there with a bunch of clothes that no longer fit him, and a photo album. I opened it, and saw this *beautiful* plan of care, describing favorite ways to soothe him, and best ways to address his medical needs. I said to myself, *Somebody obviously loved this child, and if someone else loved him, I guess we can bring him into our home and love him, too.*

"Demario was good-natured and happy, and made such progress! We got him glasses and hearing aids. He learned how to sign when he was three, and began vocalizing around his trach a little bit. Yes, he had lots of problems, but we learned so much together, and became a stronger family. In fact, he was in and out of here so many times, that I ended up at this job as their unit secretary."

I was astonished. How was it possible to be reconnected with my first Primary Care patient whose picture I had kept tucked away in a shoebox for over six years? Afraid to ask the question I really wanted to know, I inquired, "Did his family ever come to visit him?"

"No," she said thoughtfully. There was a moment of silence before she continued, softly saying, "Demario died here about a year ago, after getting an abdominal infection. It was one of many hospitalizations, but we never regretted having him in our family...and I want to thank you for showing how much you loved him, and for providing such good care, so that we could love and learn from him, too."

I will never understand the mysterious forces that led me to meet Demario's foster mother—years later, hours away, in a different role, and at the right time and place. It was such a gift. As nurses and physicians, we grapple with the ethics of prolonging a life that might become a burden or lead to suffering. Most of the time we are required to repress the experience of wondering what happens to our patients after they're transferred or discharged, never knowing whether doing what we thought best was enough, or was 'right.'

Sometimes, we manage to listen to the intuitive voices of our hearts, allowing love and compassion to lead us into the mysteries of the unknown, until the day they are untucked from the shoebox sitting on a shelf in the closet.

Karen M. Cooper, RN, BSN

Undetermined Destination

Growing up in small town America, our neighborhood was basically a re-enactment of the *"Leave It to Beaver"* show. The early 1960's were ideal years for kids to grow up feeling secure and adventurous while being nurtured by an entire village.

Our immediate village included women straight out of the *"Donna Reed"* show with their pressed aprons over lovely fitted dresses and matching high heels. On the other side of the street were the women who had careers, both out of necessity and because they desired to make a difference.

Mary Ann LeBrun was the career woman who brought the nursing profession to life for me. As an esteemed nurse in the local hospital, often working the night shift, Mary Ann seemed incredibly exotic. Our mother was a stay-at-home mom who occasionally substituted at the school so, watching a mom work full-time was incredibly fascinating to tree climbing prepubescents. To add to that aura were the tales we'd hear recalled over the fence about "catching a baby before the doctor arrived" or "sewing up the kid who'd been shoved through the plate glass window by his brother." How rapt we were hearing these stories of danger and heroism. How exciting the prospects were of earning a living rather than staying home and becoming a "June Cleaver."

Nursing was the only career choice that I ever seriously considered. My first job as a graduate nurse was in a thirty-bed hospital, *the* very hospital where

Mary Ann worked. This fine facility had busy surgical and emergency wards which became my classrooms with the "old timers" acting as my teachers. During this training time, it didn't take long for the mythical "exoticness" of the night shift to turn into pure terror and fatigue.

Our night shift staff consisted of three nurses. One was assigned the medical floor, and another the surgical floor. I, the "Newbie," was the float nurse with patients on both floors, expected to hear patient call bells through the ceiling. One night I was shaken from fatigue by a voice: "GET UP HERE!"

Heart thundering, I ran up to a room with alarm lights flashing, and found my head nurse. "*Your patient died on the toilet! I had to wait to get to the phone and call you until he was stiff enough to prop against the wall.*" *Shoot!* June Cleaver was starting to look better and better. Thankfully the fear and uncertainty of my new career didn't push me over the brink, or I'd have missed the "*Bonanza*" on the other side.

Working as a nurse gives you intimate exposure to people. Having a sense of humor has been an attribute that has served me well as I have cultivated a diverse nursing career. It is however, *reality* and *honesty* that tempered my steel and brought meaning to my chosen path.

Home Health and Hospice work were especially ripe with the people that joined the travelogue of my career. Patients receiving care in their own homes more liberally share the true essence of themselves as they act as hosts rather than as guests in your environment.

One home care hospice patient who particularly touched me was a man I visited daily, aiding him as he slowly receded from his previously robust life style. During these visits my appreciation for his crisp view of the world grew as he shared his final journey with this eager and oft times hovering nurse. One day, toward the end of his struggle, his raw candor touched me deeply as he looked up at me from the bed that entombed him and said, "You know, it's a lot easier dying than watching." How can you calculate the value of such insight?

Another patient who humbled me and showed me hidden secrets of the human spirit was the woman who, during my first visit to her home, asked me to bring her jewelry box to where she was sitting. As she thoughtfully turned each piece over in her time-worn hands, the stories of their relevance began to unfold. "I remember my grandmother wore this brooch at my wedding...This necklace was given to me by my first love..."

As the sun faded on that afternoon, the room was filled with the glint of many precious stones and cherished pieces of finery whose values were established not by their monetary worth but were measured in the memories they embodied. The brightest glimmer however, shone in the sunken face of a fading woman who once again experienced the remembrances of vitality and hope.

Could any experience be more poignant than that of holding your own grandmother in your arms as she slipped into eternity, all the while singing hymns, carols, and reciting Bible verses? This woman who had taught me about life, in her final years had been robbed of her keen mind but *never* of her sense of humor. Our family realized the gift of her presence and the honor of being taught about "the good death" along with the "true treasures" of living a good and honorable life. I wouldn't trade those moments for the world.

Today, I have arrived. I am proud to be a school nurse who, after thirty years of continuing to perfect my craft, is comfortable and capable within my world of nursing. The path to this arrival has at times been a rocky road with the destination never clear. Even though I never identified a specific career goal, my nursing journey has been incredibly rewarding and filled with experiences gleaned from nearly every corner of the medical field. These side trips through the constantly evolving medical profession have formed the nurse that I am today.

The drama that is life and nursing could never be scripted into the episodes of a television show. Who could write the dialogue for the young girl who came to me in tears early one morning, distraught over the death of her pet chicken? Trying to console her, I said that sometimes people had beloved pets stuffed at the taxidermists. Taking a deep breath she replied, "Sheesh, it was *just* a frickin' chicken!"

Or how about the day that a unique and precious child was concerned about the CPR she had just learned, wondering whether she'd be able to perform that "hind lick remover."

Another enriching element of my job is that I had the pleasure of working with my brother. One day during a Social Studies class, his sixth-graders gathered articles from our regional newspaper. The class was relatively quiet until one bright but impulsive girl finished her portion of the paper, stood and blurted, "Can anyone give me a C-Section?" Snorting mixed with guffawing could be heard the length of the hallway!

Life is filled with moments like these—moments of joy, sorrow, confusion, humor and anticipation. In nursing, as in life, if you are waiting for the "June Cleaver" moments of perceived perfection to encompass you, you'll miss the important instances of simplicity, love, acceptance and truth. As a nurse, you will see people at their very best and very worst. If you allow yourself to aid these fellow life travelers by giving them comfort or by sharing their joy, then you too will *arrive* at your undetermined destination.

Amy Nelson Knutson, RN, BSN

A Nurse's Journey:
Expectations, Hope, and Compromise

Hope: a feeling of expectation and desire for a certain thing to happen; grounds for believing that something good may happen.
Oxford American Dictionary

As a nurse, one invests one's heart and soul in the care of those in need. My journey as a nurse has been an exercise in the modification of expectation, as well as an understanding that the desires and aspirations of the healthcare team do not always match that of the patient. These differences can be the cause of great heartbreak on the part of a clinician. It is by moderating our expectations wherein we can often find the most peace, and paradoxically, the most realistic hope.

Jose was a kind, illiterate man who spoke only Spanish, had a third grade education, and signed his name with an "X." He had a history of childhood trauma, heroin addiction, alcohol use, and a track record of non-compliance. Coordinating his care—with Hepatitis C, AIDS, diabetes, hypertension, and mental illness—would be difficult. Assigned to my already enormous caseload, he would take up more and more time as his condition deteriorated. Still, our interactions were always pleasant, and our mutual affection grew with time.

Complaining frequently of abdominal pain, Jose was given medication for reflux disease and was coached about his diet. With an enlarged liver, there was little we could do to alleviate his symptoms, and we adjusted his medications on a regular basis. His diabetes was out of control, and his care was complicated with challenges related to transportation, language barriers, illiteracy, and social isolation. Luckily, he seemed to grasp the importance of his antiretrovirals—the medications prescribed to keep his HIV undetectable.

At first, I was brimming with hope and enthusiasm that Jose's diabetes would come under control, and that he would understand the importance of making good choices. Time and again, I would bang my head against the proverbial wall, reiterating my instructions on how to choose wisely. When I would check the memory in his glucometer, I would see results in the 400 to 500 range—the normal desired result being between 70 and 110.

When questioned about a high blood sugar, he would recount a visit to a friend's home, the array of desserts, and the joy he experienced in sampling them. Frustrated, I would tell him how damaging such high sugars could be, illustrating for him how blindness, amputations and dialysis were only around the corner. He would laugh and promise to do better, apparently amused by my frustration.

When Jose began to test positive for opiates and cocaine, my hopes for his long-term health were dashed. Discussing his relapse, he would say, "I just can't stay clean for more than a few years."

We would talk about addiction. He would agree to counseling, but the following week he would explain why he missed his appointment. Eventually every mental health agency in the city refused to see him.

"You know I'm disappointed that you won't go to counseling. Just because you relapse doesn't mean you can't be clean again. Let's start over," I would say.

"It just doesn't work for me. Just keep coming every week and we'll see how I do, OK?"

I wasn't happy with his responses, but I persisted in my efforts to keep him on track.

Some months later, one of the blood tests for his HIV showed that his "viral load"—the amount of circulating virus—was elevated. I called the pharmacy to see when he had last refilled his prescriptions. The pharmacist said it had been three months.

I drove to Jose's house, enraged, and demanded answers.

"I can't take those pills no more," he said. "They hurt my stomach and I feel so tired. I can't do it. No way." He hesitated. "I was afraid to tell you."

You know," I said, "those pills were keeping you alive. Your viral load will continue to rise, and then your immune system will weaken. You'll die of some infection that we could have avoided. This is crazy, Jose!"

Despite my efforts, there was no turning back, and he would never take antiretrovirals again. His blood sugars would remain high, and he would frequently test positive for opiates, cocaine and marijuana. I would sometimes tell him that I was giving up hope.

"Don't give up on me, man," he said. "I need your help. Just do it my way."

I resigned myself to Jose's modus operandi. Since his doctor wouldn't prescribe narcotics while he was using drugs, I could only advise him to stay clean so that we could control his pain, which appeared to be worsening.

When he did agree to stay clean, we switched him to methadone. His doctor took my word that Jose would not sell it, and agreed to prescribe the methadone as long as Jose tested negative for illicit drugs, which he was able to do about 75% of the time. While I couldn't control his AIDS or his diabetes, I *could* control his pain. The battle was waged on many fronts, and I began to count my blessings when I could put out a small brush fire before a wildfire erupted.

Eventually, Jose developed pain in his abdomen that would not go away. After more than seven months, he finally allowed his doctor to order an abdominal CT-scan which confirmed our worst fears: Jose's abdomen was riddled with cancer.

Radiation to such a large area was not guaranteed to be effective, and Jose suffered its many side effects. When he refused chemotherapy and surgery, we realized that end-of-life care was now our only choice.

Hospice nurses began regular visits. Jose was miserable. I would visit every few days to coordinate his care and touch base with the hospice team. We increased the methadone considerably, but Jose's pain was unquenchable.

It seemed so long ago that I had hoped to bring Jose's diabetes and AIDS under control. Where once we had hoped for years of quality living, now we could only hope to keep his pain moderately controlled as the cancer spread. Where once we had planned for him to take a vacation to visit his family in the Dominican Republic, now we could only scheme to get him into the bathroom without falling.

Writhing in pain—a catheter in his bladder, a raging fungal infection in his throat—he thanked me for all

I had done. We cried together more than once. Although I felt that I had failed, he absolved me of all guilt. He reminded me that we had done this according to his rules—not mine—and that, in his eyes, we had succeeded.

My hopes for him had originally centered on *my* agenda. My "feeling of expectation" for "something good" was based on a premise that Jose had shared my goals. I, *The Heroic Nurse Care Manager Who Saves the World* was confronted with *The Recalcitrant Patient With a Complicated Trauma History Who Wanted to Do Things His Own Way.* Of course, I was certain that *I* would win the tug o' war, and that Jose would live fifteen or twenty more quality years due to my timely and thoughtful intervention.

But that was not to be. Like so many of my patients, Jose's hopes differed from mine. He hoped to have a piece of cake at his neighbor's house. He hoped to score a bag of heroin once in a while and have some fun with friends. He often hoped that he could fool me long enough so that I would leave him alone for a few days. He also hoped to die with dignity in his own home, and he looked to me to make sure that happened.

One day, Jose told me that his brother was coming in two weeks to take him home to die. While we awaited his brother's arrival, we continued our attempts to control his pain. Care now centered on comfort, and the hospice nurses made sure that everything was done to alleviate as much of his suffering as possible. We would visit, joke about our times together, and he would regale me with tales of his Dominican childhood.

Finally, Jose's brother arrived and together they made Jose's last journey between New England and his tropical childhood home. I was sad to see Jose go, to lose that sense of closure of being with a patient until the end, but I was happy that he was choosing to die on his own terms. That brought me great peace.

Several weeks later, I called Jose's brother's home. After an interminable wait—with a television blaring and the sound of numerous voices speaking at deafening volumes—Jose struggled to the phone. We chatted for a few moments. I told him that I loved him, and that it was an honor to have known him. He blessed me before we hung up. I imagined him lying on a small bed, a picture of Jesus on the white wall, the sounds and smells of family life enveloping him.

He died a week later, and is buried in a cemetery in the small rural town where he spent his youth. I hope to visit some day, and pay homage to our friendship.

When considering Jose and the notion of hope, it is clear in retrospect that our hopes were often at odds. As a medical provider, I entered our relationship with a set of expectations and an agenda to which Jose was expected to conform. *My* hopes and aspirations—for disease control; adherence to diet, meds, and appointments—were all well and good, but Jose had other goals. He made certain that *his* hopes were realized despite the fact that he often needed to defy me in order to accomplish them.

In the end, my ultimate hopes were indeed realized, with Jose returning to his home and dying in dignity, surrounded by family and the smells of home cooking. While *my* clinical goals were often ignored, *he* was the driver of his bus, and I was admittedly merely a passenger.

Jose taught me to accept that a great deal of patient care is indeed out of my control, and I have since integrated that difficult lesson. He taught me to reevaluate my hopes, and to simply trust in my patients' choices, even when those choices reap results that I myself might eschew. In Jose's case, I did indeed choose trust, and I coupled that trust with a decision to simply bear witness as he found his own way. Thus, when all was said and done, I was able to release him with a blessing and an open heart, and for that I am eternally grateful.

Keith Carlson, RN, BSN

My Cosmic Uncle Sam

It's so strange to find myself in a situation that I can only explain spiritually. Throughout most of my life, or at least the first half, I prided myself on being sharp, sarcastic, cynical, funny. *I* was the one with the quips, the ready answers, the glass half-empty, the worst case scenario.

In June of 1986 all that changed when my three-year-old daughter was diagnosed with leukemia. Suddenly my family was plunged into an alien world, replete with its own language, equipment, customs, heroes and villains.

I was a young mother with five-year-old and six-month-old sons, and a little daughter whose ashen face and aching bones caused her pediatrician enough concern that we were immediately whisked off to the Yale pediatric ER. I'd had the reputation as a bit of a hypochondriac mom, running my kids in and out of the office every five minutes, only to be sent home with an encouraging, if not slightly exasperated, pat on the back. I remember thinking, *I told you she was sick,* just like the bad joke about the hypochondriac's epitaph.

But, truly, I don't remember thinking much at all during that period. My husband and I took turns at our daughter's bedside. I spent nights, and he would bring our baby son so that I could nurse him in the mornings. Our lives became a blur of chemotherapy, broviac care, lumbar punctures, bone marrow biopsies, vomiting, steroid craziness and stress.

We went to support groups at the hospital and at the Leukemia Society. We met Bernie Siegel—author of *Love, Medicine & Miracles*. I was angry, bitter, cynical and couldn't hear anything he had to say. Nothing and no one could comfort me.

I watched my beautiful little girl with the long curly hair go from thirty-five to ninety pounds in two years. She became a bald, bloated, cranky, needy, sick little kid. I learned to give her methotrexate weekly through her central line, oblivious to the seriousness of the procedure. We met other kids with various types of cancer, going through chemo and surgery.

In spite of my bitterness and alienation, little touches of humanity sent little green tendrils through the cracks of the wall I'd built up around me. This little girl would die without a liver transplant; that one lost an eye; this one, a limb; that one, an organ. One would never have children; one couldn't tolerate the chemo; another, the radiation.

We parents sat at meetings looking manic, like demented deer caught in the headlights. *How do we get them to take the medicine? How do we help them get through the nights without waking in terror? How do we get them out of the car when they know it's a lumbar puncture day? What do we say when they ask if they're going to die–and we know that they are?* We cried. We laughed. Although there were many different stories, our hearts ached as one.

Despite myself, my frozen pain, I spent time at the bedsides of dying children. I had a strange sort of comfort there. I began to recognize an ability to provide comfort and solace to the mothers. I wasn't afraid or uneasy.

I learned simply to be present. Where did this ability come from? To this day I still don't know.

Here's what I do know.

One fine day I was standing in my dining room feeling fed up and hurting right down to my core. I had never been a praying person—quite the opposite in fact. Suddenly I was possessed with the urge to literally turn my head to the sky and say, "If you let me keep my daughter I promise I'll give you something back." My desire to become a nurse had finally decided to announce itself.

So there I was at the ripe old age of thirty-eight with three little kids; former careers as a newspaper reporter, teacher, costume designer; a confirmed cynic; with some sort of cosmic Uncle Sam pointing his finger at me saying, *"I want you!"*

With no clue whatsoever of what I was getting myself into, I entered nursing school. I would love to say that the universe sent me little beacons of inspiration along the way, that every now and then I would turn my head to the sky, smile in a holy way and know I was doing divine work.

No, I did *not* turn into Mother Theresa. That one little moment of divine inspiration turned into two years of all too worldly perspiration. Panic attacks in the ICU, tears over a medication error, anxiety seizing my bowels in the ER were more the norm for me at the time.

But all through it, in spite of myself, that little gift would appear. Just when I would think the situation was too intense, too much for anyone to handle— the family that needed to discuss DNR (Do Not Resuscitate) in the ICU, the husband of the woman I'd just unsuccessfully done CPR on in the ER—the gift would come, and I would handle these situations with grace.

It's no surprise I went to work at Connecticut Hospice straight out of nursing school. I remember my first day walking through those big wooden doors in my white uniform as a graduate nurse. It was a moment of pride stronger than any I'd ever felt. But more than that, it was a moment of complete "rightness." I'd done the right thing, followed the path that was laid out for me when I had no clue what I was doing.

In the seventeen years since I've continued in my hospice career. I've mellowed, as we all do, and hopefully, have gained some wisdom. My daughter is still beautiful, a twenty-five-year-old woman with exceptional empathy and compassion. I've finally become certified as a hospice and palliative care nurse. Sometimes I feel exhausted by all the pain—physical, emotional, and spiritual—that I witness. When I do, I've learned to become still. To listen for that little voice that tells me I can handle it, that the gift is still there. It always is.

Liza Leukhardt, RN, CHPN

Nora

In the fall of 1961 at 3:00 a.m., I met Nora. I have never forgotten her. As a third-year nursing student, I was working nights on a medical floor, and it wasn't going well. Nights were hard. I was sleep-deprived, scared, inexperienced, and to top it off, two months pregnant—with twins as it turned out.

So far that night, I had gone in to check on a man and found him in the throes of death. That incident left me shaken and feeling more than a little inadequate. After that, I had calmed an older woman with a broken hip who'd been disturbing other patients with her incoherent yelling. Now she was at it again.

Before going back to her room, I answered a call light at the end of the hall. Inside, a thin, young woman with short dark hair, sparse from chemo, sat at the foot of her bed, tangled in her covers.

As I helped free her from her bedding, she asked for a glass of tomato juice. I hurried to the kitchen. No tomato juice. So I poured a glass of apple juice, and took it to her.

When she saw the glass, she looked stricken. "I want tomato juice. Please," she said, her voice shaking. "I crave salt, and they won't let me have any. Tomato juice seems to help." Her eyes were dark pools of pain and need.

It took more time than I could spare to find tomato juice. But what was my time compared to hers? When I brought it to her, she gulped a few swallows, calming a little. I resisted the urge to walk out of her room, away from facing her truth. Instead, I sat next to her on the bed—against the rules for nurses—while she sipped the rest of her juice and talked.

Her name was Nora, and she was dying from breast cancer. She was only twenty-five; she missed her husband and four children, including a fourteen-month-old baby; and she worried about them trying to get along without her. Her mother was helping care for the children.

She paused for a moment, then told me matter-of-factly about her surgeries and treatments. The doctors had tried everything they thought could save her—extensive surgery first to remove her breasts, later her ovaries and other organs. She'd had chemotherapy and radiation treatments. They all had failed. Now she had been moved to a private room. Her doctors visited as infrequently as they could.

What she left unsaid seemed to hover in the air.

She wanted to know about me. I said I was newly married and pregnant. She smiled for the first time, and I felt like crying for the beauty of it. We talked only a short time, but in those few minutes, we connected on some deeper level.

All too soon, I had to go. I settled her in bed as best I could and returned her empty glass to the kitchen.

After that night, I began feeling more tired than usual. It wasn't long before I started spotting. I stayed home, rested a few days, and the spotting stopped.

The powers-that-were said I could switch to dayshift, and I was assigned to a medical floor in the new wing. I went back to work, my developing twins hanging on for dear life.

A couple weeks passed before I had time and energy to stop in and see Nora. As I headed to her room, I saw her family standing in the hall. Her husband, tall and sandy-haired, looked pale and overwhelmed. He held a baby girl while two little girls in pretty dresses stood shyly at his side. A boy about two hugged his father's leg.

I spoke to them briefly before going in to see Nora. The simple navy blue dress she wore hung on her thin frame. Her body trembled from the effort of getting dressed. When I looked into her eyes, mixed with the unfathomable sadness was a spark of hope. She smiled. "I'm ready now. I'm going home."

I never saw her again.

We had shared a few precious moments before Nora's life ended and mine continued. I have always been grateful for those moments.

Marjorie Rothermel, RN

The Best Part

Margie was a grown woman in the body of a nineteen-year-old girl. The twins she carried were already mad, trying to come out before it was time. *Preterm labor,* we called it. Her adult face revealed deep lines that spelled hardship and determination. I sensed that it was life—not so much the contractions—that was responsible for her pain.

I remember how anguished I felt when she told us that she could not possibly stay at the hospital to allow the medicine to stop her pains, which were coming too fast and too soon. She had a two-year-old at home. Her mother was on drugs. Her grandmother was sick, at another hospital. And she did not want her little sister to miss any more days of high school to baby-sit. I kept asking, *"Isn't there anyone? A friend? A neighbor? Anyone?"* I wanted there to be *someone.*

A social worker came, and was quickly dismissed by Margie. I began planning, in my mind, how I could work it out to get her two-year-old to my house. But before I could figure this out, she was leaving, AMA—against medical advice. AMA also translates into "noncompliant," "irresponsible." As I met her gaze, her eyes warmed, and she silently thanked me. For trying. For thinking. For knowing that she was anything but. *Irresponsible.*

A few weeks later, Margie showed up in active labor. *Alone.* She had made it almost to term, but the babies were small, and slid easily out of her tiny body. I cannot remember their sexes, because this happened about fifteen years ago in Chicago. But I remember her in the recovery room—in our old dank recovery room, which was separate from both the labor and delivery rooms.

I was surprised to see Margie sitting up in her recovery room bed, wide awake amid a jumble of blood-speckled sheets. She was trying to breastfeed! She had breastfed her other baby, and *"he was healthy,"* she said, beaming. *"So why not these two?"* She wanted the best for her babies, right from the start.

I was privileged to help her put her baby to breast. Although she said she had nursed before, she was awkward—like she had forgotten how. Or maybe she was having trouble because of the anxiety she felt while trying to position one baby, while the smaller twin was in the nursery being monitored more closely.

After I helped her baby latch, Margie started asking me questions. *"How many years did it take for you to be a nurse? Was it hard? Do you like it?"*

I would like to believe that Margie is now raising her children to be productive members of society—perhaps even future nurses. I know this is possible, because *I* was a young single mother myself, and completed nursing school while raising my sons. My sons never joined a gang, sold drugs, or went to prison. Instead, they both went to college and serve as positive role models for other African American males. Maybe hers will too. But I cannot really say what happened to her, or to her children.

What I can say is that being a nurse, I get to meet people from diverse walks and paths. While teaching them about their health or about their illnesses, I learn *from* them. About life. While supporting my patients throughout their journeys, or even through their darkest hours, I am sometimes reminded of my own life and all its frailty. But mostly, I am amazed by the remarkable courage and resilience of the women I serve each and every day.

My life is enriched knowing that at the end of each day, I have touched someone's life in a special and meaningful way. That's the best part of being a nurse. *The best part.*

Adrienne Muhammad, MSN, NP

Nursing in the Big House

My new inmate breathed with mouth open, nostrils flaring, and using every accessory muscle in her upper body to struggle for breath through the conglomerated cement of PCP pneumonia. A forest of lead-white thrush expanded to the edges of her cracked lips. Her dark skin was stretched tightly over her cheekbones and her friable hair fell out in clumps. Thirty years old and newly diagnosed with AIDS, she had been transferred by ambulance, on day shift, from her regional jail.

At midnight, her PICC line—a special catheter placed by a physician—stopped working. She had a fever of 104.5 and her blood oxygen saturation was down to 92%. I tried using a heparin flush, but was unable to reopen her PICC.

"Your line is blocked," I said.

She looked at me blankly.

"Miss Jones, I can't get the medicine into your body. I'm going to need to start an IV."

She turned her head away toward the celadon green cinderblock wall. I returned to the Plexiglas and steel-girdered control bubble and phoned the on-call doctor.

"Start the IV," the doctor agreed, her voice muffled. I pictured her in bed. "Give 1000 more of Tylenol. No oxygen yet—and call me back in an hour."

"She's bad, isn't she?" the officer asked, nodding his head of grey slicked-back hair toward the new inmate's room.

"Yes, she's working so hard to breathe, I'm worried she just might give up and stop," I said, pouring two 500 mg tablets of Tylenol from the big stock bottle into a small paper cup.

"We're pretty well staffed; you want me to ask the Sarge to put someone in the room to keep an eye on her for you?"

"That would be great," I replied, grateful for his help in the first medical crisis of my professional career. I had passed my Boards only two months earlier, and Miss Jones was the first patient I thought might die on my watch.

I walked back to her room as the officer called the Sergeant. I poured water from Miss Jones' bedside pitcher into a small plastic cup and dumped the Tylenol in—per prison protocol—to make cheeking meds more difficult. She took the cup and swallowed the mixture of water and dissolving Tylenol without turning her head. After she showed me her mouth and stuck out her tongue in accordance with prison routine, I returned to the bubble to gather my IV supplies.

I found a tourniquet, gloves, alcohol pads, Tegaderm, tape, and blue pads, but no linking hubs in the nurses' station. "I have to go down to the supply closet; we don't have everything here," I said putting the supplies into a clean emesis basin as an older, female officer arrived.

She related to the inmates with a maternal dynamic. A good officer either yelled at the inmates daily or not at all. The officer in the infirmary control bubble was a jokester, using humor to keep the inmates in line and never showing his frustration. In prison everyone picked a persona—inmates, officers and staff alike. Successful inmates found a social role such as grandma, drama queen, or underling, and stuck with it.

"So you just need me to sit with her?" the officer asked.

"She's angry at the world; she's not talking to any-one. I think all you *can* do is sit," I said.

"What do I do if she stops breathing?"

"Call 10-52 Code Blue on the radio and start CPR till I can get here. I just need to get some IV supplies," I said, as she furrowed her brow. "I'll be right back."

"Okay, honey—I'll do my best while you get your things together," she said, patting my arm before walking to the isolation cell.

On my way to the supply closet I passed the main pharmacy where two LPNs pulled the pill line all night for the eight hundred inmates who took a.m. meds. At the other end of the building, a psych nurse watched over the acute mental health unit. Four nurses. Twelve hundred inmates. No IV team to call, nobody to fall back on if I couldn't get the stick.

Walking down the hall, I remembered my tour when I came to interview for the position of night nurse in the infirmary. I was fascinated by the world of the prison, a little city embedded in the countryside. During nursing school I worked at a big university hospital as a nurses' aide. I wanted something different after gradua-tion.

Well, you've got it, I thought as I used the big, tawny brass Mogul key to open the supply closet. *You wanted the challenge of autonomy—here it is.*

While my fellow new grads were doing competen-cies on infection control, I was at the Department of Cor-rections. Learning about locks and keys, and how to respond if taken hostage. My friends from school were training in months-long mentorship programs. I had two weeks shadowing a woman who I found crying in the break room before every shift. She showed me how to connect the arcane IV links and hubs, but neglected to show me where things were stored.

Searching the shelves, I spotted the links, grabbed a handful, and hurried back to the infirmary. In the bubble I used *another* set of keys to unlock the IV-start needles and syringes from a steel box within the locked med cart. Each needle and syringe would have to be signed out and accounted for before the next shift arrived.

I put everything into a mauve basin and walked toward my first independent IV start as a registered nurse. During my Emergency Department practicum, I'd started two or three a day. But that was a few months ago.

The steel door of the isolation cell was propped open and the officer sat in a chair beside Miss Jones. "Am I going to be in your way, honey?" she asked.

"No, I'll start over here," I said, walking to the opposite side of the bed. "Now, Miss Jones, I'm going to start an IV on you so we can get your medicine going again."

She didn't respond as I put on gloves, placed a blue pad under her arm, and applied the tourniquet. A nice "Y" formation popped up on top of her hand. I decided to shoot a 20 gauge straight down the Y and cleansed the skin. The veins fattened and the alcohol dried as I opened the Tegaderm, tore my ritual three long thin strips of tape, and opened the syringe package.

I pre-filled the syringe with saline, then hooked it to the connecting link.

"Okay, Miss Jones, here we go," I said, unscrewing the plastic sheath from the IV needle base and sliding it away from the metal needle. "Give me a deep breath."

I breathed. She did not. "Big stick now," I said as I slid the needle into her vein. I felt as though I was watching myself from the other side of the room—seeing the flash of blood in the chamber and pushing the catheter forward until I could retract the needle. Her crimson blood spilled down her hand and soaked into the blue pad as I plugged in the link, released the tourniquet, and pushed the saline.

After securing my masterpiece with a strip of tape over the IV hub and a V-formation over the link, I cleaned the blood with an alcohol pad, and covered the site with Tegaderm. The adrenaline in *my* blood made me feel shaky as I hooked up her antibiotic and watched it drip—counting the drops and adjusting the flow.

"Nice job, Stassen," the officer said, as I cleaned up.

"Thanks. I'll be right back to check her vitals," I said.

Miss Jones continued staring at the wall.

Walking back to the control bubble, I felt like a nurse in the Wild West, nursing on the edge. No longer shaky, I felt like a gun-slinging sheriff walking though town after killing an outlaw. I signed out the needles, returned the unused ones, grabbed the vital sign equipment, and hurried back to the cell.

Miss Jones' temperature was 102. Her oxygen saturation hovered at 93%, and she seemed to breathe a little easier. I called the doctor again, and released the officer to another wing.

After three days, Miss Jones' IV infiltrated and she was switched to oral antibiotics. The following month, her CD4 counts responded to antiretroviral therapy, and she finally began talking to some of us.

"My fiancé gave me this disease," she said. "I wasn't some 'ho."

Used to her silence, her abrupt words startled me. I thought her first words would be something more mundane—like, "Dinner was terrible."

I paused. "I'm sorry," I said. "But you're doing really well now. You responded quickly to the first combination of medication the doctors tried—that's a good sign."

She made eye contact and nodded before turning toward the wall.

During my assessments throughout the following weeks, we talked about living with HIV. We focused on role models like Magic Johnson, who'd been publicly positive for thirteen years. "When you see him on TV he still looks good," she said.

After two months of living in the infirmary, she began participating in a school program. While helping her with her math homework one day, she said, "That's your mark. I've got the mark of Nurse Stassen on me." Putting her pencil down, she pointed to the small scar on her right hand. "I was so angry that night, wasn't I?"

"You were going through a lot," I said, smiling.

"I didn't understand you were helping me—I didn't know what was going on. Some people would have caught attitude back, but you've always been nice. I wanted to thank you for that," she said.

I felt like I might cry. I wanted to tell her she'd left her mark on me, too. The night I took care of her was a turning point for *both* of us. She proved to me I was up to the challenges of the job. I felt proud of every pound of weight she had gained. But I knew the Corrections mantra, "firm, fair, and consistent." Just as with children, I could never show favorites.

"I was just doing my job," I said, and patted the scar on her hand before leaving her cell.

Sara Stassen, RN, BSN

An Old Soldier Heads Home

As boys of sixteen, we high school buddies were always on the lookout for someone to buy our Friday and Saturday night beer. Across the bridge in the woods near the Old Soldier's Home, Ollie had built a hut made of sticks, where he camped out, away from the Home, during the warmer months.

One night the Bosley brothers borrowed their mom's car, knowing that Ollie, ever alert for a little cash to buy himself a bottle, was in the woods. When Buck Bosley spotted Ollie gathering firewood near the edge of the forest, we flagged him down.

We cut a deal before Ollie, along with his over-whelming odor, got into the car. Rolling down the windows we drove back across the bridge to the liquor store. Ollie had his bottle and we had our beer. Let the Good Times Roll! We dropped Ollie off near the woods and parted ways.

The next time I saw Ollie was when my buddy Sean and I, for our senior Social Studies project, went downtown to interview the homeless. We learned that Ollie had once been a farmer. One summer an angry twister blew in and he lost his wife, his children, and his farm. His story saddened me.

We also met a thin little fellow named Gary, who spoke fondly of his Forest Service work fighting fires and harvesting timber in Montana. I asked if he was related to a former major league baseball player with the same last name; he boasted that he was.

Two years later, I spent some time wandering, down and out in cities far from home. I hitchhiked, camped, ate in soup kitchens, and lived on people's couches. My initial attempts at family life ended up on rough and rocky shoals. I found myself alone in our deserted home when the words of the Apostle's Creed came into my heart and began to grow. After a bit of time, my heart led me to the Catholic Church.

When I returned from life on the road, I settled back in my home town and graduated from nursing school in 1977. As a new nurse, my first job was at the county Detox Center where homeless alcoholics came to dry out. We nurses made sure they didn't die of the D.T.'s while they were sobering up. From time to time Ollie would come in. Along with him was little Gary, often brought in by the police. A few times he had some rough D.T.'s and we nearly lost him.

After several years at the Detox Center, I went to work in adolescent drug treatment. We worked with kids addicted to drugs or alcohol, and their tattered families. Within a few years I had gotten worn down by these adolescents and went looking for something a bit slower paced.

I began working with the elderly at the Old Soldier's Home, where farmer Ollie and little Gary were residents. My wife, whom I had met at church, introduced me to the ways of Saint Francis and I volunteered to lead the Rosary for a group of men and women at Elder Home, another nursing home. Connie, an old Polish woman and a Secular Franciscan, was one of its ailing patients. One day when I went to take her to the chapel for Rosary, she said she was feeling too sick to go. I asked if there was anything I could do for her. She asked me to get some brown scapulars to offer to those at the Old Soldier's Home who were near death.

I went to the Catholic store and picked up a half-dozen brown scapulars, along with information about offering them to the dying. A few weeks later, Connie lost her own battle with cancer.

It wasn't long after that that little Gary, whom I'd met as a teenager so many years ago, began a major battle with cancer. A lot of water had gone under the bridge since my high school Social Studies project and his years of revolving doors at the Detox Center. I went to Gary's bedside and offered him a scapular. Too weak to talk, he nodded his acceptance.

As part of the scapular ritual, there was an added blessing for the dying person if they would listen to a prayer and kiss the scapular. I offered this to Gary as he lay there, breathing with difficulty. He nodded "yes" with as much enthusiasm as a dying man could muster. I held the scapular to his lips and he gave it a kiss. I was the privileged eyewitness to what seemed to me a miraculous conversion.

The next morning, we knew Gary was going to die. The hospice chaplain came in and got to know Gary a bit through sharing Bible stories with him. The on-call hospice nurse asked if Gary had any relatives. I knew of only one—his nephew Phil of whom he'd spoken with much animosity. The nurse called Phil, who said he'd come if Gary wanted him. We asked Gary, and he indicated "yes."

Just before noon, Phil arrived. In the presence of the chaplain Phil and Gary were joyously reconciled with tears bedewing the cheeks of all. More restful now, Gary slowly slipped into a place where he no longer responded to us. Shortly, with his grateful nephew at his side, Gary made his final passage to the Father.

And so by some deep mysterious logic, Jesus had been using Gary and me over the course of the forty years we had known each other. If my work means nothing more, that one day with Gary, and the influence of Connie, has made it all worthwhile!

William Robert Moore, RN

Why I Thank Them

After thirty years in nursing, I still had boundary issues. I wanted all my patients to remain friends long after discharge so I could continue to monitor their progress. As I hurried from my car toward Rodrigo's front door, I wondered—again—if I should have bought a gift to celebrate the fact that he was finishing six months of daily Directly Observed Therapy (DOT).

Monday through Friday on my way to work at the Health Department, I'd stop at Rodrigo's house. He'd open the door with a smile on his face and a bottle of water in his hands. After handing him a plastic bag with his tuberculosis meds inside, I'd stand and wait while he swallowed his pills. On most days I'd ask in my terrible Spanish how he was feeling; his response was always so fast and long that I'd pick up only a few words here and there.

This special treatment began after Rodrigo had gone to the county hospital the previous summer. He was barely able to walk, his legs severely bowed by childhood rickets. In the pre-surgery work-up, they'd discovered active tuberculosis so instead of the hoped-for surgery, Rodrigo left the hospital with medication that left his fingers numb but slowly eased his cough.

Rodrigo, who was not a legal citizen, had a history of substance abuse and incarceration. Because he couldn't be trusted to take his medication, he was deemed "non-compliant," which called for DOT. Since his house was on my route to work, I began each day at his front door by 7:30 a.m.

Early on, I'd learned from the medical case worker that Rodrigo didn't live in this house. It was owned by relatives who let him sleep on a sofa in the garage. Most mornings he was dressed and waiting for me at the front door, but a few times I'd had to go looking for him. I'd make plenty of noise and then pretend I didn't notice him pulling on his pants and limping across the patio. He'd duck into the back and rush straight through the house to the front door, while I quickly rounded the porch to ring the bell one more time and pretend that I'd been waiting there all along.

On this last morning, Rodrigo shocked me when he opened the door as I came up the steps. Proudly sticking out his hand, he said, "I know that I'll never forget you, mama." We shook hands, both of us smiling at the other. The sounds of traffic and lack of time prevented any meaningful conversation, so I wished him well and left him with my card.

I waved as Rodrigo watched me drive away, and I realized I was going to miss seeing him each morning. Driving to my office, I thought about what he'd said. His comment made me wonder if all those mornings I'd made small talk, asked about his family, encouraged him to eat right, to follow up with his doctor, and to keep his clinic appointments made more of an impression than I had thought.

Public health nursing has an image problem. We don't save lives in dramatic ways as the ICU nurses and we generally seem unappreciated in the larger health-care picture. Physicians see their patients in offices or in hospital clinics and are the generals who get most of the attention in the war against disease. They test, prod, scan, determine the problem and plan the attack.

Eventually the patients are discharged with prescriptions in hand, determined to get better or possibly not even understanding what is wrong—or worse—maybe not even caring any longer. We all hope they have families that can help them, but often they lack any support system at all.

Every morning across the country, public health nurses set out to put doctors' plans into action so that the doctors can move on to their next patients. We see what they don't, what they can't, or even what the patient doesn't want them to see. We visit patients in their own homes, encountering problems doctors might never envision.

Because the patients don't eat right they won't heal, but all they have is a toaster oven or they eat most meals at the McDonalds down the street. They've been placed on insulin for their diabetes but can't afford the syringes, or they lack transportation to the pharmacy that doesn't deliver and peripheral neuropathy prevents them from walking that far.

Their hypertension is out of control but they can only afford to take their medication every other day. They wonder whether it will still work, but are too embarrassed to ask their doctors. And even though doctors can smell it on their clothes and know their patients are less than truthful when they say they've stopped smoking and drinking, they don't see what we see—the ashtrays filled with butts, or trash cans filled with empty beer bottles. They may suspect, but the fact is that we face it head on every day and still maintain hope that we can make a difference.

There is too much disease, too little time and not nearly enough compensation for physicians to make house calls these days. In truth, the patient in the office waiting room is often very different from the same patient sitting in his own home.

I learned this years ago from Rudy, an elderly Italian-American man with congestive heart failure. For years he had come to my office with his wife so I could measure his blood pressure and assess his condition, which never really improved. His feet grew so swollen that he wore only slippers. Each month he grew more short of breath and, as his health declined, his complaints grew and I ran out of responses.

Rudy changed physicians several times, saw many specialists, and tried every possible medication for each of his complaints. I'd listen to his chest, weigh him, examine his ankles, and follow up with his physicians who were as frustrated with him as I was. Labeling his chart as "probably non-compliant," I tried to listen patiently, but I dismissed many of his complaints as bids for my attention.

One day Rudy's wife called to say Rudy was requesting a visit. I must admit I was curious, and because I hadn't seen him in a while, I agreed to stop later that day.

It was a glorious late spring afternoon, nearly dinnertime when I finally arrived. I rang the bell and through the window Rudy's wife motioned for me to go around back. Although they lived in the suburbs, they had built what looked like an Italian villa, complete with a white stucco house. On a hill behind was a small patio shaded by a grape arbor where Rudy was sitting in a lawn chair. He wore a thin jacket despite the warm weather and a nearby table held a glass of red wine. The breeze rustled the leaves as the soft sunlight shone upon his bare head.

"Hello there!" he called to me in his thick accent, a big smile on his face. "Thank you for coming. Welcome to my home. I want to tell you something," and he waved expansively to another chair. "CARMELLA, BRING HER A DRINK!" he bellowed, and she rushed to bring me an iced tea.

For the next hour, Rudy smiled broadly as he told me about his life. He talked about the restaurant in Little Italy he had owned, how he had met his wife there, about the children he'd raised and the home he'd built. I heard in detail about the church he attended, the clubs he joined, what to plant in my garden and how to select a tasty wine. He'd had a good life. He seemed to be telling me that although he knew he'd complained for years, he was grateful I had listened.

I saw him then for what he was to others—a successful businessman, a loving father, a gardener, and a man who'd been full of life for so long and bitterly resented the illness that finally limited him. As the afternoon turned to evening and the air began to cool I helped Rudy return to the house, impulsively giving him a hug before I left. A few weeks later, Carmella came to my office. Her shoulders shook as she told me that Rudy had died not long after my visit.

Though I'd been a nurse ten years or more, that afternoon was a turning point for me. It changed the way I thought about how I practice. Every patient has a life outside of what I'm easily able to see and it's my job never to forget that. My thanks go out to Rudy, Rodrigo and to all the patients since who have reminded me that nursing is much more than drawing up plans of care based on symptoms. Unless I can take time to understand them as individuals—as more than a syndrome or a collection of complaints—I will never be successful at helping them. I'm still surprised when they thank me, because, without them, I would never have learned what the textbooks failed to teach me.

Thanks to Rudy and all the other like him, I'm able to believe that I have made a difference in many people's lives. I still begin each shift looking at my patients, wondering, *Will* you *be the one I reach today?*

Christine Contillo, RN-BC, BSN

An APRN's Journey

I knew as a young girl that I wanted to be a nurse and work in mental health. Being a "people watcher," it was very easy for me to bond with other people. When I announced to my family that I wanted to be a nurse, the responses were mixed. *"Why not be a doctor or a teacher?" "But nursing is such hard work—and all those bedpans and things."*

My parents' goal for me was to attend college, a goal they could not reach because of the Great Depression. Florida State University had a new academic BSN program, so my parents and I could both achieve our goals! In 1957 I graduated from FSU with a baccalaureate degree in nursing. My nursing career was interrupted by marriage and the births of three children, but I was able to work in various areas on a part-time basis.

In 1972 while working on an acute care mental health unit, Ann—an RN colleague—and I attended a two-year "Group Work" class at a nearby psychiatric hospital. We incorporated our new knowledge in group therapy sessions for our patients, only to find that after discharge, patients often waited months before being seen at the overwhelmed community mental health center. The need for continued group therapy was obvious. *Why couldn't we do that?*

In order to establish our own mental health group therapy practice, I took a graduate level course taught by a masters-prepared RN: "How to Establish Your Own Business." We presented our plan to the hospital psychiatrists, emphasizing it was a means of adding a needed service to our patients. They agreed to support our efforts.

Ann and I—after consulting an attorney—agreed on a simple partnership. We obtained a city business license, purchased liability insurance, opened a joint business account, and designed the necessary forms and stationery. Since insurance companies would pay us only if a supervising psychiatrist signed the insurance forms, we worked out a contract with each psychiatrist.

Getting started, we knew we had to "prove" ourselves. This realization was validated when many of our first patients were distinct challenges.

A local church agreed to allow us to meet in a large room which usually worked very well, but there were a few surprises.

Our meeting room linked the sanctuary and the education building. One evening in December, when our group was very small, we were discussing whether the members were benefiting from such a small group—and should we continue? Unbeknownst to us the church choir was getting ready to rehearse in the sanctuary. At the very moment the group made the decision to continue, the choir started singing the Hallelujah Chorus! Laughter *is* good medicine!

Another time a bridal party paraded through our meeting. The more sobering event was when a casket was brought through the room. We survived it all, and each event stimulated the group.

I soon realized that in order to advance clinically or administratively, I needed to obtain my masters degree. In the early 80's, I became a Psychiatric Clinical

Nurse Specialist certified by the ANA Credentialing Center (ANACC).

With the growth of our practice, we graduated to a psychiatrist's office complex—with two groups, and then three. Since a change in the law allowed APRN's to bill directly to insurance companies, we no longer were required to have a physician's signature. We were now *independent practitioners*.

At this time I was also the assistant director of the hospital mental health unit. Our practice was growing, business was booming, and we often had "psychiatric borders" who would spend their days on the mental health unit and sleep on the medical units.

When I read about a new role emerging for masters-prepared psychiatric nurses, Psychiatric Liaison Nurse, I called the medical facilities in our area to see if they had one. None did. I read everything I could find on this which was very little, but enough to help me design this service for our hospital.

The Psychiatric Liaison Nurse would, per a physician's order, see patients anywhere in the hospital, do a psychiatric nursing assessment, write a note in the Progress Notes (where only physicians wrote at that time), and would continue to see the patient if requested. The Liaison Nurse would recommend that the patient be seen by a psychiatrist if necessary.

I presented the proposal to the Vice President for Nursing, who accepted the proposal, contingent upon the Psychiatric Department's approval.

I prepared carefully for the Psychiatric Departmental meeting—emphasizing that this was a way to reach patients with mental health needs who could easily be overlooked in the busy hospital. The psychiatrists approved it on a "wait and see" basis. The department chief informed the medical staff of the new service and we were off and running.

Again, our first patients were true challenges, test cases as we saw them. We received referrals to see brain damaged patients, chronic schizophrenics, delirious patients and patients the nurses weren't able to control. We never said "no" to a referral.

My role as a Psychiatric Liaison Nurse included supervising two other nurses. We practiced independently as a nursing service sponsored by the hospital, and it was wonderful to feel the respect and appreciation for our added service.

After our first year, we sent a satisfaction survey to the nursing and medical staffs. The responses were informative and positive. Our service was now engrained into the fabric of the hospital, and accepted by the psychiatrists—perhaps because we filled a need which brought more patient work to them.

To acquire even *more* marketable skills, I took a two-year course in Organizational Development through the National Training Laboratories. This prepared me to assess problems experienced by organizations similar to those experienced by humans. Later, a two-year course at the Juran Institute prepared me to be a Continuous Quality Improvement (CQI) Group Facilitator/Trainer.

The hospital asked me to create a Performance Improvement Program based on the Juran model to train hospital staff to effectively participate on CQI Teams. Another masters-prepared RN and I did just that and became facilitators for the teams. At this point, as an APRN I was therapist, administrator, teacher and facilitator. It felt very good. I also became a Magnet

Recognition Award Appraiser for the ANA Credentialing Center. All my years of experience in the above areas proved invaluable.

In 1999 I retired from the hospital, but continued my private practice and my work as a hospital appraiser for ANA. Though I retired from the Magnet Recognition Program in 2006, I continue to enjoy my private practice as an APRN.

What have I learned from this journey? I've learned that dreams can come true if you're willing to study hard, work hard, love what you do, be professional, abide by the rules, be responsible, be a little gutsy, and be able to laugh at yourself.

Anne Scott Fredrickson, MSN, APRN,BC

Nurses in Bald Places

The patients in Room 652 and 653 couldn't be more different. What they do have in common is something they lack: they're both bald. Room 652 is a woman with a glioblastoma...a stealthy brain tumor that has a way of killing fast. She's fifty seven, same as me.

"The doctor says I'm history," Teea says softly, without affect or apparent fear. Her humor is deceptive. I bet she'd bribe, threaten or supplicate all creatures, medical or otherwise, two-legged or eight, who promised her even one extra week. She wants to live so bad she could scream to the heavenly rafters, but she doesn't, at least not in the hospital. She behaves calmly here.

Each of her three daughters is distinctly striking, as beautiful as Teea herself, even though radiation therapy fried the hair right off her head. She only has curly clumps above her ears now, like a clown.

"I'm thinking of having them bronzed," Teea fusses with the clumps, "so Mom can put them on the mantle above the fireplace, next to my baby boots."

Teea's oldest daughter studies primates somewhere in Africa, and came home two days after her mom got the lethal diagnosis. The middle daughter's in the Air Force, training to be a pilot. The youngest lives nearby and is expecting Teea's first grandchild. All three are at the hospital as regular as rain.

Teea figured the lion's share of her own parenting duties were behind her, and she just wanted to sit back on some padded chaise lounge, drink a nice Australian red, and watch her daughters do what they do best. She wanted to be the audience. Applaud, witness, detach if she could. But not die.

Room 653 has a bald head too; clean-shaven after smashing into a windshield of a stolen car he careened into oncoming traffic. He's seventeen.

Both of the men in the Toyota van he ran into died right there on the highway. A father driving to the Honolulu airport with his visiting son, a young and popular volleyball player who'd finished his college career with 731 digs. His handsome, grinning face was all over the news that night. Come to think of it, he was shaved bald, too.

Even though the wreck was mid-afternoon, room 653's blood toxicology was positive for methamphetamines, benzodiazepines, alcohol and cocaine. The accident damaged his brain even further than his habits.

He's skinny. Street drugs had suppressed his appetite's voice for some time, tricking him into imagining he was not just high, but full. At first glance his body looks like it belongs to an emaciated, dying old man. Closer up it's easy to see his sculpted muscles are like hardwood.

He wears a too-large plastic diaper and his limbs are tied to each corner of the bed so he doesn't hurt himself or us nurses. He yells constantly. Most of the noises are unintelligible, but he does seem to know three words: *sit, no, how.* The way he says "sit," we're suspicious it's a mispronunciation. "No" is sometimes "nnnnnnnnnoh", and other times "nooooooooooh." More often than not, "how" is a long repetitive sound with several syllables, like a chant. The emphasis is usually on the "ow" portion, leading us to wonder if he's in pain.

The nurses give him analgesics even though they don't seem to help. They give the meds because it makes them feel like they're doing something useful. They give them because his yelling drives them crazy.

No one visits him. There's a note on his board that says, "Grandma and Noni called to say they love you. Get well soon."

He's a hard one to like. The nurses give him feedings of a thick sweet-smelling liquid the color of dirt, pushed into a gastric tube tunneled into his stomach. They clean him up and put mitts on his hands so he doesn't chew his own fingers or scratch himself bloody.

For someone tethered in four places, room 653 is all over the bed. In the two weeks since his accident he's rubbed his heels raw. His diaper hangs low on his angled hips, and most of the time he's able to squirm out of it. Last week he gave a night shift nurse a nasty bruise on her upper arm while she was trying to talk him down, to comfort him. He bit through the wrist restraint and swung at an enemy none of the rest of us can see.

Teea and I have had a few good talks about God and destiny and the source of wellness. That kind of human intimacy is what I live for.

Today, however, I decide to spend a few of my precious moments in room 653. I don't feel much enthusiasm for it, but my job as a pain and palliative care clinical nurse specialist includes assessing suffering. Yesterday when I called him by name, he stopped yelling. But when I left he just resumed, no matter how many tranquilizers or opiates the nurses gave him. If my presence can quiet him down, it will at least give the staff a reprieve.

I roll a computer into his room to do some chart-
ing. "Brandon," I shout over his shout. He makes full-on
eye contact and stares like a baby does, not quite in
focus but very intent on something he sees. "Brandon,
do you have pain?"

"No," he says, as nonchalantly and clearly as if
we'd just resumed a lucid conversation over a cup of cof-
fee, then he goes silent. He stares at me, he stares at the
walls, he stares into thin air. Every once in a while he
tracks something across the ceiling, as if a shooting star
has flared above him.

I tell him about things. I tell him I want to make a
movie of him, to show high school kids what really happens on drugs. I figure the diaper might get them. I ask
him how it could be that some people want to live with
every fiber of their spirit, and others seem to dare death
to come find them. Brandon doesn't argue or inter-
rupt. He lies there in total silence. I don't have much
time.

"Brandon, I have to go." He stares at my lips as if
he hears something remotely familiar and unnerving,
like the pulsing of a troubled mother's heart.

Heading toward room 652, I see Teea's husband
Robbie leaning against the wall outside her door. His
eyes greet me with a grief as dense as the door itself, and
a question that has no answer.

I lean up against the wall next to him. He tells me
that the hardest thing about Teea's diagnosis is the
helplessness. A high school biology teacher, he likes tan-
gibles. He tells me the ground beneath his feet moves
like sand, and he cannot find purchase.

"Noooooooooooooh," shouts Brandon. I follow
Robbie into Teea's room.

"Honey," Teea looks up to see her husband's help-lessness. "Go sit with that young man next door." Rob-bie leaves willingly, taking his question with him.

Hob Osterlund, APRN,C

More than Making Beds and Emptying Bedpans

"It's not as if you're working as a proper nurse anymore," she said, arms folded, eyes glaring. "When was the last time you made a bed?" she asked.

I was teaching a clinical update, to a group of community and hospital nurses. The woman in the front row had been tutting and rolling her eyes at almost everything I said. I had seen her look of disapproval when I walked in. Not only was I a man, but I wore my hair in a ponytail.

At first I just stood there, surprised and dismayed at her comment. If *that* was all she thought of nursing—the physical tasks of making beds and emptying bedpans—then she had a poor view of our profession. Although it had been nearly ten years since I made a bed in my professional role, not for a single moment had I considered myself less of a nurse.

When I qualified as a Registered General Nurse (RGN) in the early nineteen-nineties, nursing was in the midst of a heated debate about the "Extended Role." Nurses were assuming many of the roles traditionally associated with doctors, such as cannulating patients, planning hospital discharges, and operating clinics as independent practitioners. Many nurses resisted these changes, insisting we concentrate on the "basics of nursing care." This apparently boiled down to making beds, washing patients, and checking vital signs.

I believed as nurses we should be looking forward and developing our profession. Instead, I found working in hospitals stifling. Nursing was still task-oriented, and the hierarchy continued to demand nurses defer to doctors. Where was the holistic care that had been talked about so much during my training?

In 1999, my waning enthusiasm was restored when I moved out into the community. There I found my second wind, working with a group of community nurses. We managed our own caseloads and had time to give to our patients. We were involved at the heart of the assessment and planning of our patients' care—working closely with doctors and drawing together many other healthcare professionals. *This* is what I had come into nursing to do, to nurse people back to their best quality of life, instead of rapidly moving them toward discharge on a never-ending conveyor belt.

I have experienced many roles in the community—community nursing, telephone triage nursing, out-of-hours nursing—and always with a high degree of health education involved. There is no greater pleasure to me than imparting information so that people can make informed decisions about their health, empowering them, rather than rushing in and saying, "*I* can do that for you."

Currently I work in audit and training, educating those who provide patient care. Though my patient contact is low, my role is important. I give patient care providers the most up-to-date information for them to perform their jobs, ensuring that quality service is delivered.

In addition, five years ago I expanded my nursing role into journalism. I write regularly for *Nursing Standard, Nursing Times*, for a national men's health publication, and I've recently begun contributing articles on health care to a London newspaper. I wish more nurses would discover journalism; our society seems hungry for informed writing on health matters and is not always well served.

When I qualified as a nurse—so long ago it seems—I never envisioned my career taking the path that it has. My highest ambition then was to become a nurse tutor, thinking that was the only way I could develop as an educator. I am no nurse tutor. But this, to me, is the joy of nursing, the variety of roles that are available.

While my nursing path has led me into education, there are a plethora of opportunities for today's nurses. Opportunities that several participants in that clinical update stayed around to discuss after the critic stomped out at the end of the session.

As for her—what did I say? I simply said, "There's more to nursing than making beds and washing bottoms."

Drew Payne, RGN

Of buck teeth, nebulizers, and the Tooth Fairy

A fifteen-minute nightmare: It was a quarter past three in the health room and I had a child who had been there since 2 p.m.—a little third-grade girl who had a fever. No one was available at home to come get her.

At 3:15, she vomited across a huge area of the health room in front of the asthma inhaler cabinet.

Simultaneously, two students from phys. ed. came in saying, "We need our inhalers!" I checked them with the stethoscope, jumped over the vomit, and got the inhalers for them.

At the same time, there was a kindergartener in the bathroom, standing in a puddle of urine because of a bladder accident, naked because he had taken off his wet clothes.

Meanwhile, buses were rolling into the parking lot.

As I escorted the sick child out to the bus so the driver would know he had a child with a fever, the rest of the staff were waving to me from the parking lot, "*Come here, Maggie! Come here, Maggie!*" A child had hit his head in phys. ed. and I had to make a decision: Should we put him on the bus?

In assessing his pupillary response, I noticed something was not quite right, so I got his mom to come get him. He ended up being transferred to the hospital with swelling of the brain.

That was one of the worst quarter hours of my career. Luckily, it's not all like that.

I became a school nurse because, as a child, I had what we call buck teeth, or an overbite, to the point where my brothers called me "Bucky Beaver."

My parents could not afford the orthodontic treatment that I needed, but our school nurse, Marie Kelly, took a picture of my smile and sent it to our state capital in Albany, where they provided the orthodontia that changed my life: I could smile, not cover my mouth with my hand, and not be afraid of being teased.

Another reason I became a school nurse is that I enjoy long-term relationships, and when you work with a family, you may have a relationship as long as 12 years by the time all the siblings have finished school.

I've worked in hospitals, but there, it's a very short relationship.

The thing I like the most (and that I didn't expect when I became a school nurse) is the response I get from students. When I go into classrooms, I like to use drama. When we do dental hygiene, I dress as the Tooth Fairy. Later on, they'll see my costume and say, "There! We *know* you're the Tooth Fairy!"

And I'll just say, "Oh, no. We just look alike, and I let her leave her costume here."

Since I started as a school nurse 23 years ago, many things have changed in our student population—drastically.

Some of the most pronounced changes are in technology. We have students who, 20 years ago, might have been in specialty care centers because of their disabilities—a school for the deaf or the blind, or a children's rehab institute.

Now, because of technology, we have user-friendly equipment that allows children to attend their community schools.

It's not unusual to have nebulizers going in the health room. We have students with cerebral palsy in motorized wheelchairs. We're doing bladder catheterizations, tube feedings, insulin pump monitoring.

So technology has brought students who would not have been in their community into the school— where they should be. But it's taken us a little time. We're scurrying around to catch up with the needs of those students.

And that's one of the many reasons why it's so important that every school have a qualified school nurse.

You really need someone who can see the difference between a harmless bump on the head and a concussion.

Maggie Compton Beall, BS, MA, RN,BC

Warm and Fuzzy

When I became a nurse forty years ago, it was one of the few options for women of my generation. I have loved almost every nursing job I have had since then, and have worked with many great nurses.

After a year's retirement, I started over with a new and challenging job. Nothing in my career: public health nurse, school nurse, hospital nurse, nursing home nurse, home care nurse, private duty nurse, mental health nurse, American Red Cross volunteer nurse, and college nursing instructor has challenged me as much as my new job. *Prison nurse.*

The warm and fuzzy feeling you receive knowing you have done something to make a patient's life easier is so rewarding. I remember times when I made a difference for someone and times when another nurse made a difference for my family or for me.

In prison nursing, you really have to stretch to find warm and fuzzy moments. At first, I didn't feel the nurses in the medical unit were very "caring." When an officer called to say an inmate was in pain, the more seasoned nurses often responded that they would go see them much later—when they passed meds.

Not me. I would run down to the appropriate cell block and give him something for the pain. That's part of what nursing is about, right? We make life more bearable for those ill and in pain. But what about the person who caused his own pain because he punched a wall; or was bitten when beating a smaller, younger inmate; or developed *another* staph infection, after receiving his twentieth tattoo? Inmates tattoo each other all the time, even though it's forbidden.

What about prisoners who call you names and threaten to sue after they've refused to come out for meds—because *now* their health is suffering? What about those who come in again and again because they have addictions, poor judgment, or mental illness, and are so unable to understand even basic life tenants that they can function only in an institution?

You may think it's hard to like these inmates. Some of them are murders, rapists, addicts, sociopaths, or child pornographers. Many are products of dreadful backgrounds, surviving each day the best they can.

One of the hardest things I have had to come to terms with is to like them, yet maintain a basic professional relationship. You want to mother the young, clean-cut man who is always cheerful and polite and comes to med pass, but then he and several others beat up a smaller or younger person just to prove they are tough. You may find you respect the man who is calm and quiet and doesn't abuse the use of PRN medications, until you learn he has been abusing and intimidating others; or he raped a twelve-year-old; or he killed his friend while on drugs; or any number of other heinous things.

In the end, we nurses are professionals, and that has gotten me through some sad, angry, and draining times. My fellow nurses advised me it is better not to know why these people are in prison, and now, after having done this job for eight months, I find they are right.

I am a nurse. I will pass medications and bind wounds with care. I will take time to be cheerful, to give smiles and sympathy to everyone. I will listen to their stories and symptoms because sometimes no one else does. I will do health teaching as much as possible. I will advocate for the downtrodden and mentally ill. If someone is depressed or anxious, I will refer him to mental health staff and let him know I care.

I am a nurse—a vocation I love. I help others, whether they know it or not. *Sometimes*, they do know. They say, "Thank you; you helped me." So there are some warm and fuzzy times after all. After forty years, I still believe I can make a difference.

Barbara H. Toenyes, RN, BSN

A Call to Pastoral Nursing

Some call this inner voice Conscience, some call it God. I call it Spirit. Today I am a Pastoral Nurse. It's more than my employment; it is my calling, my vocation. This change occurred when I listened to my inner voice—that guiding force within.

For twenty years I worked in a corporate environment where I became discontented with the work, disenchanted with the corporate structure, and disturbed within my soul.

So, in 1990 I left the corporate job to train as a Massage Therapist. Unfortunately, misleading self esteem challenges had convinced me to question my abilities in mathematics and science. However, after I completed the required algebra, anatomy and physiology classes, I recognized not only was I capable, I could excel.

One day a fellow student suggested I look into the nursing program. I did, and three years later, began working as a Geriatric Nurse in a primary care clinic. In addition, I worked as the Director of Residence for the Edgewood Retirement Center. During this period I began my studies for my Master's Degree in Nursing—my goal was to become a Nurse Practitioner.

Meanwhile, my husband needed to move to Missouri that fall to complete his ministerial studies at our church headquarters. Thinking that we would need to supplement our income, I suggested that I stay and work as a Nurse Practitioner during his time in Missouri.

I was on a new journey—seeking more autonomy in my work—but as this journey continued, I began experiencing doubts. *Did I truly want to be a Nurse Practitioner? How would this career combine with being the wife of a Minister?*

Nurse Practitioners are trained to treat patients and families with the same standard of care as physicians. My professors desired to see the role grow and gain more respect among other health care providers. I wasn't happy with where the academic program was taking me, and began to realize that the program was only part of my preparation. I wanted something more holistic—something more spiritual than dealing exclusively with medications, differential diagnoses, and treatments.

My good friend and nursing mentor was a Parish Nurse. As I listened to her talk about her work, I felt a calling to this area of nursing—engaging the spiritual with the physical. But instead of heeding the call, I dug my heels in to complete the program and begin work as a Nurse Practitioner.

Then one day, down on my knees and begging for guidance from Spirit, I received a very clear message. I heard, *"Sit still."* Several times during meditation I heard these same words, but chose to ignore them.

Instead, I piled things onto my plate. I continued both jobs, working thirty to forty hours each week, and changed from being a part-time to a full-time student. Though I was discontented with the strict philosophy of medicine I was hearing, I was anxious to get started as a Nurse Practitioner.

Spirit was telling me to sit still, but I resisted. Resisting Spirit is like pushing against a wall. As I pushed, I began experiencing physical phenomena. My muscles ached. I felt pain in my knees, then my shoulders, and eventually in every joint in my body.

On graduation day in June, I was so stiff and sore I could barely move. Since my husband's celebration for the first tier of his Seminary program was the same evening, we agreed to go to our respective ceremonies. My mother and a good friend accompanied me to my graduation dinner. I was physically unable to drive and was exhausted by the time I returned home.

Finally, my doctor diagnosed my illness and started me on medications. My pain began to subside. I now recognized what was going on—my illness was related to my resistance to Spirit.

I began to listen to my inner voice in earnest. The message came less than a week later. It was, *"Wither thou goest."* I interpreted this to mean I was to accompany my husband to Missouri and become part of his ministry. I didn't know how that would be accomplished, but I followed in faith that it would.

When we arrived in Missouri, I was too weak to take a job. I spent my time praying and reading the plethora of spiritual literature from the church library. I remembered the calling to Parish Nursing, and discovered that the Parish Nurse Certification Program was offered at a hospital less than twenty miles from our home. While my husband finished his ordination path, I enrolled and became a Parish Nurse. I was led to a wonderful Parish Nurse mentor with whom I worked for one year. After my husband's ordination, we moved back to Michigan to begin working as a ministry team.

Today I embrace the calling and duty that are mine. I serve as the Pastoral Nurse alongside my husband in our new and growing church in California. My duties include—but are not limited to—counseling congregants on how to blend their spiritual beliefs with their physical issues. We discuss nutrition, disease processes, courses of treatment and medications—and I encourage them to seek and explore all options. I advise them to pray first. We discuss their comfort levels in various situations, and I offer guidance on how to listen to what *their* inner voices are directing them to do.

I give thanks each day that I learned to listen to Spirit. I am grateful that I continue to reinforce this lesson for myself and for those I counsel as I joyfully serve as a Pastoral Nurse.

Michaelle Washington, RN, MSN

There Is a Time to Die, But No Time to Cry

Monday night, she was smiling.

After I gave her an enema, she smiled. After I gave her a heparin shot, she smiled. After I repositioned her, even in obvious pain, she smiled.

I don't think it was because she was elated with the things I did for her. It was just because there was nothing else to do. She spoke only Hindi, and—when she did talk—I had no clue what she was saying.

So, she smiled.

I had to call her daughter in the middle of the night when she refused the second enema. I explained the situation before passing the phone. Then, *she* talked to her daughter for a few minutes, passed the phone back to me, nodded and motioned me to continue. Again, that smile.

Granted, that the sad results came back that night, and the hateful tumor was labeled malignant, but still. She was not one of those patients who reeked of death. She was weak, yes. But dying? That did not even cross my mind when I left Tuesday morning.

When I came back Tuesday night, I was a little surprised that her name was not on my patient list, but I was not concerned. I thought they had moved her to a basic unit, or worse, to ICU.

Then, they told me she had died.

I wanted to cry. Out of shock, out of empathy for her very enthusiastic daughter who filled me in with every little detail of her mom's life in the few minutes that we chatted. Out of the sense of sadness that overtook me—the kind that daughters share when they lose their moms.

I wanted a moment. A minute or two maybe, just to be sad, because that's how I felt. Sad.

Unfortunately, my job didn't give me the luxury of that moment. To make matters worse, there was the annoying irony. A couple of my coworkers who sensed I did not take the news very well tried to dismiss the idea of grieving—even for a moment—by saying, "Come on, May, she was better off going anyway."

Granted, that was true. But was it wrong to grieve anyway?

No, it wasn't wrong. It was just that there was no time. *Literally*. Four patients waited for me, all needing my undivided attention. There was blood pressure to be stabilized, a confused patient to be kept safe, a psychotic patient to be watched, an unresponsive patient to be monitored—whose children huddled in the corner of the room, crying in frustration and fear. Clearly, the last thing all these people needed was a teary-eyed nurse, crying over a patient who was no longer there.

So I bit my lip, started my night with the same smile I usually start with, and ended it physically tired and emotionally unfinished. I hadn't found that moment to grieve. Not until now. It may sound overly dramatic that I am taking that moment now, a long time after the fact. But I am. Here, now, where I have the luxury of time.

It's not that I do not welcome death. It is the uncertainty of when it is coming that I wrestle with. Especially with people who seem to have so much to live for.

It's not that I do not understand others' "death-doesn't-get-to-me" attitude. I do, and have reacted that way plenty of times. It's just the fact that sometimes, we are left with no other choice but to wear that "I-couldn't-care-less" façade because we don't have time to do otherwise.

Nursing is such a conflicting job sometimes. We are expected to be human and sensitive so we can take better care of our patients by feeling what they are going through, for their sake. And yet, we are also expected to detach ourselves from our emotions so we can take care of our patients and make intelligent decisions, *also* for their sake.

When I think of nurses who have done this for twenty years or more, I wonder how they continue to cope with conflicting expectations. I wonder how they maintain balance and still be good nurses. You know, the kind of nurse who is not immune to human emotions but who does not get overwhelmed by them, either.

Lucy May J. Colegado, RN, BSN

I Pass on the Torch

December 5, 2008: It is three o'clock in the morning and I am wide awake. This is my first night as a retiree. After twenty-one years, I am no longer a public health nurse. *Did I do the right thing? Will I regret it? Will it still please me when I'm sixty four?*

I live in southwestern Ontario and this decision did not come lightly. For the past seven years, I have loved my work, but have hated the one hundred km (sixty mile) commute to and from Walkerton during storms. After facing many fearful commutes over the years, I realized I didn't want to do that anymore.

My path to nursing was unusual. In 1975, I was married, had two children—aged ten and eleven—and an unemployed husband. I realized the $2.35 per hour I earned as a pharmacy clerk would not provide the security we needed, so I visited Canada Manpower to find out what retraining options were available. The results showed that I could do college level work, but the only feasible local program was nursing. That was it. No Florence Nightingale and the lamp—just a need to survive and do well by my children.

In 1977, after graduating from Georgian College in Owen Sound, Ontario, I was paid the handsome sum of $6.00 per hour as a "casual float team" nurse. I remember being thrilled, knowing that I was earning ten cents a minute *and* was on the road to financial security.

I had enjoyed being a student, but it didn't take me long to discover that I *loved* being a nurse. As a float nurse, I enjoyed the mystery of patient care—the wonder of each new baby, the excitement of the emergency room, and the privilege of providing comfort to dying patients and their families. I worked with so many wonderful nurses and, throughout my entire career, I tried always to return their kindness by welcoming new staff.

A year later, when the first opportunity for full-time work became available—on a psycho-geriatric ward—I accepted it. I thought it would be the opposite of what I really enjoyed, but I grew to genuinely like it. I worked in other mental health areas and, it was odd, but wherever I was, it soon became my favourite place.

Then, divorced and in my late-thirties, I realized that if I wanted doors to open for me, I needed a degree. I applied to, and was accepted by Ryerson University in Toronto.

After graduating two years later, I joined public health. It felt like this was what I had been waiting for my whole life! I loved health promotion and quickly moved from being a general staff nurse to becoming an AIDS educator.

It was a heady time. AIDS was new; there were patients to help, fascinating people to meet, and so much to learn. There were great opportunities to speak at meetings and conferences. Everyone, it seemed, was looking for an expert.

In 1990, I remarried, moved back to the country, and worked again as a public health nurse. I started to focus on injury prevention in 1996. My career was cut short by the E-coli crisis in Walkerton. This was not a clinical experience; this was a *lived* experience. Thus, I took early retirement in September of 2000 to take care of myself and my ill husband.

By the next spring, our health improved and I approached Grey Bruce Health Unit in Walkerton about a health study on the water crisis. I was invited to set up the infrastructure, which was a time-limited process. I came for a few weeks—and stayed seven years.

In the sunset of my career, I had the unique opportunity to coordinate a program funded by the Ontario Neurotrauma Foundation. The "Stay on Your Feet" program, pioneered in New South Wales, Australia, focused on helping older adults prevent falls.

I assembled a team of dedicated professionals, and together we set up initiatives: awareness and education, media promotion, community skills development, home hazard reduction, and policy. The grant ended in 2005, but there was overlap into 2008. We created a medication interaction fact sheet, developed community and in-home exercise programs, and produced theatre troupe performances—which continue today.

So, my path *through* nursing has been varied. Along the way, I met so many true professionals. I was blessed with some managers who truly believed in giving the workers the tools to do the job, and then letting them do it. I was inspired by people like Dr. Robert Conn, former CEO of SMARTRISK; and by nurses and other professionals who gave their all to design and implement programs to help people avoid the trauma of injuries.

Now, I am a consultant for the Ontario Neurotrauma Foundation. But I will never stop being a nurse, just as I will never stop trying to prevent falls. On my last day of work, my program manager took me out to lunch. Another patron tripped on a small step and fell. After she was cared for, I spoke with the staff about putting a strip of a different color on that step to increase visibility and prevent falls.

Nursing has been very good to me. In addition to the financial security that I was looking for, it has given me so much more. And my wishes for future nurses? That you love what you do. That agencies offer working conditions that are conducive to safety and job satisfaction. And I wish, too, for a strong emphasis on prevention, so less funding is needed for treatment.

Nursing is an adventure, and I pass on the torch. Celebrate the art of nursing.

Marguerite Oberle Thomas, RN, BScN

My Heart Sings

I first discovered my interest in the medical field after earning a microscope at the tender age of ten. Back then, I was a big fan of *Mad Magazine*. The inside back cover regularly featured ads promising all sorts of great prizes—for simply selling greeting cards and wrapping paper door-to-door. I filled out the form, taped on my quarter, and sent for information.

Shortly thereafter, I began my very first sales job—collecting orders from my neighbors and my friends' parents. I earned several prizes that summer, but my most prized possession was the microscope with the shiny little mirror. It sat in my bedroom window—where the light was just right—and opened up an exciting new world to me.

I think I was always interested in biology. I can remember dragging out the old World Book encyclopedia and turning to the frog dissection and to the human plates. I would study them forever—flipping each plate back and forth to survey the wonders inside.

My foray into medicine was further developed when I received those dreaded braces while in junior high school. I enjoyed the staff at the orthodontist clinic despite the torture, and was always bugging them about the tools they used, how they made the molds, and whatever else I found that tweaked my interest. I decided to write my career development paper on orthodontia that year. When my braces were removed, I glued them onto a poster board as part of my presentation complete with head gear (Ack!), wax, rubber bands and other torturous devices. I learned that an orthodontist could make $100,000 per year—in 1979!—and all I could see was dollar signs. *This* would be my new career choice, I decided.

Then, in high school, I *loved* biology. I distinctly remember my first dissections; the smell of formaldehyde and—because we didn't wear gloves back then—the way it made my fingernails grow. My instructor was delightful and engaging, and I stayed with her for three years. She encouraged me to pursue nursing and was responsible for my admission to the Future Medical Personnel (FMP) club.

During this time, I often had dinnertime discussions with my parents about career options. My mother was a stay-at-home mom while my dad was a typical middle class father, working forty-hour weeks at the local aluminum plant—where he was one of hundreds of employees. He had started there as a journeyman machinist soon after he and my mother were married. He served in the Vietnam War, and then returned to his job and completed thirty-eight years in a smelly, greasy machine shop.

I once asked my father how he could go to work day in and day out at the same plant, and perform the same tasks. I will never forget his words. *"I never said I liked it."* He explained that it was a good job with good benefits; it allowed for stability and provided for our family. His father and brother worked there, too, and he said that providing for one's family was more important than job pleasure.

It was right then and there that I decided to be a nurse someday. My father asked me to explain my decision—which was easy to do. Nursing would allow me to work with different ages groups in a multitude of settings, in the community and even beyond our borders. I could move from one area to another, further my education in many different specialties, and never have to worry about being out of work. I could work at the bedside in a hospital. I could work at the bedside in one's home. I could work in a school providing care to children and have summers off. I could work in a clinic. My options were endless, but I would still be a nurse. It would prevent me from boredom—from working in the same place for thirty-eight years, facing the same people, the same work, day in and day out.

Then, I met a boy and everything changed. My life took a detour.

A husband, house, and two children later—my baby a mere fifteen days old—I returned to school to pursue my nursing career. Initially, my goal was to work in the operating room, but during my clinical experiences, I found other areas equally exciting.

Becoming a registered nurse was one of the happiest moments of my life. I was proud of my accomplishments and the detour made this all the more meaningful. Graduating with honors brought self-esteem which had been sorely lacking. With two toddlers in tow, I set out on my new career path, ready for what life had in store for me.

I landed a job working in the local hospital on the day shift—unheard of for a new grad at that time. I quickly trained as charge nurse and was enjoying my new life, and great pay. A neurologist asked me to work with him. I had never considered working in a doctor's office; I thought that was a place reserved for medical assistants and nurse wannabes. The promise of weekends and holidays off sounded nice, as did the salary and bonus options. I worked with him for five years.

Throughout the years, I have also worked nights, worked in intensive care units, managed medical clinics, sold medical equipment, and worked as a case manager. The latter satisfied my desire for patient contact, while keeping my latex allergy at bay. During this time, I discovered I had a special knack for management and organization.

I started my current consulting firm shortly thereafter and my life has never looked better.

Nursing is an incredible profession. We are consistently ranked number one in the Gallup polls as the most honest profession. We provide the caring touch, soft words, encouragement, empathy, and yes, we also provide medical skills. We teach others how to live longer, healthier, and happier. We are a powerful bunch.

When my father was diagnosed with advanced stage renal cell carcinoma, I was on hand, as the family nurse, to offer what assistance I could. My family thanked me over and over, and I didn't understand why. I hadn't *done* anything. Sure I had made a few calls, explained some procedures, collected and reviewed some test results, but that wasn't really nursing—or was it? I soon learned that indeed this is a part of nursing and we take it for granted.

We have so much to offer and sometimes it is the simple things that our patients really need. We are instrumental in helping others prevent disease, maintain and improve health; we teach others to be good health care consumers; and we share our knowledge with the next generation of nurses.

We should encourage others to become nurses, all the while explaining that this is a tough course. Burnout is a real possibility if you consistently give of yourself. It's difficult to deal with the demands of life and death while completing the obligatory paperwork and carrying out the orders of the physicians, but the rewards we reap are worth it.

Support and advocacy are two of our principal strengths as nurses. In today's health care environment, it is more important than ever for nurses to have a voice. We must use the strength and power that we often forget we possess.

Lift up and encourage one another. Find what makes your heart sing, and do it.

Victoria Powell, RN, CCM, LNCC, CNLCP, MSCC, CEAS[II]

On BEING a Nurse

Why am I a nurse? Because I don't know how to BE anything else! Oh, I am a woman, a wife, a lover, a mother, a daughter, and a sister. I am an athlete, an artist, a gardener, and a volunteer, but above all, my BEING is a nurse.

When asked, even before entering elementary school, "What do you want to be when you grow up?" my answer was always, "A nurse." Okay, so for a short time I thought maybe I would be a veterinarian, but I came back to my BEING. I could have gone to medical school, but doctors don't spend nearly enough *time* with their patients, and that was important to me. I could have gone to dental school, but dentists don't have much opportunity to *talk* with patients, and that was important to me. I needed to go to nursing school so I could *make a difference* in the lives of those I cared for. That was really important to me!

As I reflect on the nearly thirty years I've been a nurse, I struggle to find a bad time or experience. I have only twice thought about leaving nursing, but as I look back on both those situations, they became opportunities for me to grow and change within my profession. I didn't leave nursing and actually after each incident became more passionate about my BEING. There were mistakes made, assessments missed, moments of cowardice, and patients and families who didn't like me. Each of these became opportunities to learn and to not be afraid.

No other profession has such a diversity of roles—populations across the life span to care for, clinical opportunities from preventative care to critical care, advanced practice clinicians, nursing and hospital leaders/managers, educators (basic to doctoral), business opportunities, travel, and research. Where else can one have the opportunity to hold a baby as he takes his first breath, or hold the hand of an elder as she takes her last? I have become as skilled at delivering bad news as I have of good news. I use my caring to diffuse anger as well as to sit quietly and BE.

I have made a difference in more lives than I know and that is good. I am humbled and thankful for being so blessed. My two wishes are that I will continue BEING a nurse until I die, and that more people will come, BE, and stay in nursing.

Helen N. Turner, DNP, PCNS

A Reprieve

"Were you the one who called the ambulance last week when I was so sick?" she asks, as I prepare her meds and take out my stethoscope and blood pressure cuff.

"Yes, it was me. You sure didn't argue, that's for sure." I continue to rummage through my things and arrange the tools of my trade.

"I guess I could have died, huh?" She looks at me sort of dreamily.

"It was pretty likely, but we weren't about to let that happen, were we?" I respond, looking up from my tasks.

"I dunno. I barely remember what happened."

"You had thrown up before I arrived. Then, as I took your blood pressure, you grabbed the bucket, got down on your hands and knees, and vomited over and over again. Do you remember that?"

"Yeah, I guess so. The people at the hospital were so nice, especially once the transplant team had me on their floor. I hope that liver comes soon. I'm getting pretty sick."

"You still wear your beeper day and night, right?" I ask.

"Oh, yeah. I wouldn't trade that thing for all the methadone in the world."

"Good. Now—you have a low-grade fever today. What shall we do?" I put away the thermometer and other supplies.

"I'll call a cab and go to the doctor's office to get checked out. I really don't want to go to the hospital again if I don't have to."

"Promise to go?"

"Yes, I promise."

"I don't want them to have to scrape you off that floor again if I can help it." I rise to leave.

"Thanks alot. I really appreciate it."

"Hey, you're doing the hard work. I just stop by and check in." We shake hands. "See you Wednesday, and get to the doctor's office! And no Tylenol! Your liver can't handle it."

"Yeah. See you then. I'll go, don't worry. Thanks."

Last Wednesday I started my day with a bang, sending this poor soul off to the ER—dehydrated, feverish, end-stage cirrhosis working its horrible magic of visceral implosion on multiple organ systems. A new lease on life seems to have been granted, or at least a reprieve of sorts. This patient—and thousands, if not millions, like her—walks the thin line between life and death, waiting for a life-saving organ transplant as millions of viable organs are buried beneath the earth or consumed in the fires of crematoria. What a morbid waiting game indeed.

For now, another brush fire has been stomped out as the cirrhotic fire in her liver rages on. It is truly a race with time, and even the hoped-for outcome of a freshly transplanted liver cannot deliver the promised revitalization of health without a large degree of uncertainty and risk. I have seen what havoc organ rejection and infection can wreak. If life waiting for a transplant seems rough, the other side of the surgery is certainly no picnic.

Still, I could leave that house today secure in the fact that one more sunrise has arrived for my client, and yet another opportunity presented for continued life, however challenging. Yet another instance to think to one's self, *"There but for the grace of God go I."*

Keith Carlson, RN, BSN

Reflections Throughout the Years

As a teenager in the 1960's, I heard the message, "Ask not what your country can do for you; ask what you can do for your country." My biblical upbringing taught me, "Do unto others as you would have them do unto you (Matthew 7:12)." These challenges influenced my career choice. As a naïve eighteen-year–old, I entered a three-year diploma program to become a registered nurse.

I was one of a class of 160 aspiring young women. In those days, career goals were limited. The cultural norm of the day was to find a suitable husband and have a family, but the times were changing just as much as we were.

The Women's Liberation Movement arrived. Birth control pills afforded freedom without worries. Equal opportunity became a right and an expectation.

Three years to graduation seemed a long time. Yet, as I look back, those years became the foundation of my nursing career. Later generations born in the '60's, '70's and '80's cannot appreciate how dramatically nursing has changed. Gone are the days of glass thermometers, rubber sheets, wooden wheelchairs, and metal bed pans.

After graduation, I was hired to work as a staff nurse in a mixed critical care unit of twenty-eight patients. At that time, there were four beds to a room. One room, reserved for the most critically ill patients, had four cardiac monitors. There, each bed was equipped with a glass manometer to measure central venous pressure.

Three months later, I was transferred to the newly opened cardiac care unit to work night shift. This specialized area was set aside for the sole purpose of treating patients who had sustained myocardial infarctions. Bedside cardiac monitors—the new technology—tethered patients to their beds by long cords. Bed rest was the order of the day to protect heart muscle. Bathroom privileges consisted of cold metal bed pans and urinals. And *no cold water*—for fear of heart damage.

A PVC—premature ventricular contraction—was the enemy and spelled possible doom. If a patient had two or more in a row, we called the doctor and parked the code cart outside the patient's room.

In the 1970's and 1980's, cardiac care advanced with the introduction of angioplasties, intra-aortic balloon pumps, swan ganz catheters, and open-heart surgery. Intravenous controllers and portable bedside monitors became the accepted standard of care. I attended three critical care courses, which taught me how to read continuous EKG telemetry monitors, how to interpret the wave patterns of swan ganz catheters, how to perform cardiac outputs, and what an a-line and swan reading would tell me about my patients' hemodynamics. I entered the world of pre- and post-open heart surgery. I monitored ventilator-dependent patients and acute care individuals who required continuous renal replacement therapy.

Despite all these challenges and adventures, I yearned to expand my knowledge more than bedside nursing would allow. In my early forties, I entered a

Bachelor of Nursing program. Seven years later, in 1997, I achieved a lifelong ambition—a college degree.

But, why stop? Two years later, I entered a Master of Nursing program and in three years I became a Certified Family Nurse Practitioner. While most of my peers were contemplating retirement, switching to part-time work, or remaining in stagnant jobs, I retired from the bedside and entered the world of advanced practice nursing.

A cardiologist hired me to assist him in his private practice. In addition, I entered academia and became a part-time instructor at both a private and a community college. Despite these professional and academic challenges, I felt intuitively that I had not really found my true professional calling.

After three years, I received a recruitment letter in the mail. A privately-owned company was starting an outpatient methadone clinic in my local suburban community. Though the idea sounded intriguing, I wondered, *"What do I know about drug addiction and methadone treatment?"*

Two months later, I was hired.

Now, three *years* later, I have finally found professional stability in this semi-rural setting. All the knowledge and expertise I acquired over the years have led me to this place. I manage patients who are addicted to heroin, cocaine, synthetic narcotics, benzodiazepines, and marijuana. Many have been through psychological traumas, were raised in broken and dysfunctional families, or have made poor peer choices. They suffer from depression, anxiety, insecurity, and even homelessness.

As I reflect on my career, I realize all the opportunities I have experienced as a nurse. My educational experiences led me to non-profit hospitals, for-profit clinics, private homes, publicly-funded outpatient clinics, a private office, and a prison. I have been a part of living history in health care by witnessing team nursing, patient-focused care, critical care, and step-down units. I have had the opportunity to participate in a Magnet hospital survey. I survived, and again am witnessing the "nursing shortage."

I met patients and individuals who left lasting impressions. I remember the eight-month-old boy who was burned by his mother with cigarettes. I remember the twelve-year-old girl who battled leukemia when no cure existed. At an age when most pre-teens are excited about life, she died in her parents' arms. And I remember the thirty-year-old female who died of asphyxiation because she was afraid to go to the dentist. I witnessed the beginning of life at birth and the end of life at death.

I visited a state sponsored school where twenty- and thirty-year-old Down syndrome adults had dolls and stuffed animals beside their beds. I toured one of the last Tuberculosis sanitariums. I lived with patients in a state mental health facility for three months, where one of my teenage patients had murdered his own mother.

I have come to know colleagues who have stayed with me over the years. I have been nurtured by seasoned professionals and now, *I* am the mentor. My best friend is a forty-something nurse whom I met twenty years ago. We have watched our families grow, have attended school together, and have even shared in the deaths of a parent and a brother. Along the way, we have mentored each other. Now, this dear friend has her doctorate in nursing education.

As nurses, we should realize that one life can truly make a difference. Just like the movie *It's a Wonderful Life*, where would our families, our patients, and our peers be if we were not part of their lives?

I am proud of the nursing profession—which now opens doors that in my generation were only dreams. We can travel the world, work in all kinds of settings, and even own independent practices. Today those are not just dreams. They are realities.

I am a nurse and the doors are wide open.

Joanne Whary MSN, FNP–BC

Nursing is about the Contribution You Make...Whether You Know It or Not

Working for a world-renowned consulting company was very important to me. I had relocated to a large city, had started a consuming and challenging position in my firm, and was making the best money I had ever earned in my life. But as the second year was nearing its end, the company began discussing downsizing. Only thirty years old, I asked myself some hard questions. *What did I really want to do with my life? What could I do with my life that would mean something to me—something that would give me a sense of pride?* The nice car, new suits, challenging work and daily visits to the gym were wonderful, but I felt I was missing something important. I was missing something essential that would make me feel I was not just *living* life—I was making a contribution to it.

Answers in that job were hard to come by, but I went searching for them anyway. The answer came in a form I was not expecting. I decided to do some volunteer work—and not just *any* kind of volunteer work. It had to be something difficult that would help me learn things that were not within my comfort zone. I chose to be a hospice volunteer.

There are many hospice stories highlighting why this work has such a profound effect on those involved with it. One particular person changed everything for me. She was the only patient who died the day I went to visit her. She was the only hospice patient I ever cried about—before and after her death. I cried not for her, but for her family—the only family I was alone with throughout their worst time of grief, need and loss—and for me. I was afraid that I would not be up to the task of helping them cope with their loss in a calm and caring manner, when it counted the most.

I *did* manage to assist, guide and support her family that day—in a reassuring way that surprised me. In the end, it was this patient who stuck in my heart and mind when I decided that signing up for nursing school was the next step in my life.

After three years and much studying, I began my nursing career on the oncology unit of Saint Joseph's Hospital in Atlanta. Nearly every night driving to work, I was scared to death, worrying: *Will I be faced with something I don't know how to handle on this cancer and medical-surgical floor? Will I make a mistake—with medications or in judgment? Will I remember everything I've been taught and put it to good use?*

Then, there was the night I took care of a patient's family in a way I never knew about until long afterwards. The DNR (Do Not Resuscitate) patient was entering her final hours, her breathing slowing, her pallor deepening. When I met her family, her son and husband began questioning me. How long did she have? What should they expect?

As I finished my assessment of her, it became clear that I needed to sit with this distraught family and explain what was happening. She had a very short time left, I explained. I went on to gently outline what physical things would happen to her, what I would do for her comfort, and what they could do—including saying goodbye, telling her they loved her, holding her hand, or whatever else made them comfortable as she passed away.

It was a very busy night, but I hurriedly worked through my other duties in order to spend every possible moment with this dying woman and her family. Inevitably, yet peacefully, she died several hours later. I hugged the son and his father as I cried with them, encouraged them to spend as much time as they needed with her, and eventually left the room to call the chaplain and to complete all the necessary procedures.

There have been multitudes of patients and families since then, but to say that I thought of this specific woman and her family would be insincere. I try to be present to all my patients and their families—and always with the attitude that I will do the best I can to help and comfort them—whether that means encouraging a therapy, helping a patient swallow a medication, or holding a hand until it is time to say goodbye.

Years later, something very extraordinary happened. I was completing paperwork at a nursing station when a man approached and started asking me personal questions. Had I worked on a cancer unit in the past? Had I been on the night shift? Was my name Stephanie? The latter surprised me, but I thought he may have read my badge.

As we talked, he said that his father was in the hospital. He told me his mother had died during the night shift when I was a new nurse, and that I had been there to help him and his father cope when they did not know what to expect during her passing. I was shocked, skeptical—wondering if all the complimentary things he was saying had really been in connection with his family and me. But as he continued, the hair on the back of my neck began to tingle as it sometimes does when I know I am hearing an absolute truth.

He went on to quote nearly verbatim the words I had used to comfort them—since it had been a pivotal point in his family's life—and he remembered nearly everything about it. I *was* the nurse who had helped them through the worst time of their lives. He said he had been looking for me *every time* he came to the hospital after that date—to thank me for the time I'd spent explaining and comforting them in their worst time of need. *And the conversation with my patient's son took place eight years after his mother died!*

I have been a nurse for thirteen years now, and I will never forget that family or their story. I have remained in nursing for reasons very similar to what happened in that dying woman's room that night. No matter how scared, or how much doubt I may have about my nursing skills in any given moment, I have always known I have one great ability. That is to be present for the people who need me, whether to answer questions, to hold a hand, to give a smile, to say a kind word, or to be there for someone's final moments. I learned that long ago with my hospice patient, and it has carried me through to today.

Nursing is about *being there*—most certainly to deliver medications, advice and instructions. But nursing is also about the things that are important to everyone—and sometimes intangible. Once upon a time, I searched for that something that was missing—a way to contribute to the world around me. I might not always be in my comfort zone, I might not always remember everything I am "supposed to," and I might not always have all the answers. But in finding meaning for my life, another absolute truth was uncovered: you may not always remember all you say and do for the patients and their families as they come in and out of your life and nursing practice—but they *often* remember you.

In my quest to go beyond just living life, and in my selfish desire to be "good enough," I've managed to accomplish things I never thought I would or could. Nursing has helped me relate with those around me in more meaningful, essential and often, truly spiritual ways.

Stephanie A. Lopuszynski, RN, BSN

The Notebook

I searched the hall closet for Christmas wrapping paper. Instead, I found a foot-high stack of 8 x 10 spiral notebooks. Curious, I pulled them down from the shelf. They were assignment notebooks accumulated over eight years of working for Hospice. I had forgotten about them since most of our documentation now is done on the computer.

Almost every home health and Hospice nurse has maintained some sort of notebook which is part planner, part tracker, part to-do-list, part memory, and part CYA. The good old seventy-page spiral notebook worked perfectly. It tracked my time, mileage, names of family members, names of pets, reports to doctors, and brief notes for my documentation and for my next visit. This system worked well for me. I use a smaller notebook now to jot down things I want to remember—a quote heard, a song, bits of poems, and things that touch my heart as I go about my work day.

I opened the first notebook and found the Prayer of St. Francis of Assisi taped to the inside cover.

Lord, make me an instrument of Your peace.
Where there is hatred, let me sow love.
Where there is injury, pardon.
Where there is doubt, faith.
Where there is despair, hope.
Where there is darkness, light,
And where there is sadness, joy.
O Divine Master, grant that I may

Not so much seek to be consoled as to console,
To be understood, as to understand,
To be loved, as to love;
For it is in giving that we receive.
It is in pardoning that we are pardoned.
And it is in dying that we are born to eternal
life.

I start each work day with a prayer. This prayer is very meaningful to me, because the Catholic hospital where I worked more than forty years ago used it. Prior to each change-of-shift report, we nurses recited this prayer together. This set the tone for our work day.

Below the prayer was an index card listing frequently called phone and fax numbers. In the pre-cell phone days it was easier to have these numbers on hand rather than cluttering my memory.

Pat G. was the first patient in this particular notebook. I still remember her well. She had advanced lung cancer and her doctor told her that she had two to three months to live. I met her two dogs, Reno and Rudolph. Reno was a Rottweiler and Rudolph, a Great Dane. Both were really big dogs.

I am not a dog person and asked if we could put them in another room. Pat said she wanted them to get to know me. She suspected there would be a time when she would not be able to answer the door, and I would have to let myself in.

I looked them over rather nervously. They in turn eyed me warily, especially Reno. Rudolph finally sniffed my feet, then walked over to the other side of the room, curled up, and went to sleep. Reno stayed next to Pat protectively. I asked permission from them both to take Pat's temperature and blood pressure. Reno allowed my assessment without any barking or growling. He remained attentive, but I think he sensed that I was there to help Pat.

The dogs tolerated my visits and allowed me to enter the house without difficulty. As Pat became weaker and bedbound, Reno would lie next to her bed and I had to step over him. I never chased him out of the room; he was part of her family. Pat said when she got to heaven she wouldn't have to step over big dogs anymore, but I was sure there would be dogs in *her* heaven.

I saw her on a Friday before my weekend off. I sensed she wouldn't be there on Monday. I arranged for twenty-four hour nursing care and made sure she had enough medication before kissing her on the cheek. She grabbed my hand and said, "You promised I wouldn't be in pain when I died. Don't stop the drugs."

I assured her that she had enough medication in the house. She asked for a priest to visit because she wanted to make her peace.

She did die that weekend. The family asked the nurse to go to the liquor store to honor Pat's last wish that her family toast her off. The nurse said *she* couldn't do that, but she would stay while someone in the family went to the store.

Pat had talked freely about her death—what she wanted and what she didn't want. I learned a lot from her. Reading the notebook brought back the memories of Pat—her courage, her strength, her sense of humor, and her dignity.

I had looked for wrapping paper. Instead, I found a treasure chest in a stack of notebooks.

Joanne Cherry, RN

What If He's an Angel?

Some years ago I had the honor of caring for a patient who forever changed the way I viewed myself and the way I practice the art of nursing. While his time on this earth was short, every nurse who cared for him was enriched by the experience.

My relationship with this very small patient, named Gabriel, started before he was born. The doctors had informed his parents early in the pregnancy that their child would be born with a birth defect that was not compatible with life outside the womb. They were offered the opportunity to terminate the pregnancy and avoid the physical and emotional trauma of a full-term delivery. They declined the offer.

I met Gabriel's mother when she was admitted to the hospital to have her labor induced. She was an incredible woman who had spent most of her pregnancy dealing with a reality few will ever have to face. She explained to me that she had been given the opportunity to love and care for her child in the only way possible, by providing an environment that would permit him to live. She knew it was anticipated that he would not survive his first day of life. During those precious months she had loved and cared for him, knowing that their time together was short. Soon after finding out about his problems, she had named him after the archangel Gabriel.

Gabriel's delivery was anything but routine. He surprised the doctors and nurses present by entering this world kicking and screaming. Hours turned to days,

days turned to weeks, and still Gabriel struggled to survive. During this time I had the opportunity, as his primary nurse, to share him with his mother, caring for him during the long nights that he spent in the Special Care Nursery. I spent countless hours talking to his mother as she rocked her precious angel late at night or in the wee hours of the morning. For a newborn, Gabriel did amazing things. He laughed, cooed, and blew bubbles. He charmed all of us and we knew that when he died, his footprints would remain forever on our hearts.

When he was almost three months old, Gabriel began a steady decline. He was no longer gaining weight and sometimes he would stop breathing. We all knew that the end was near. On his last night with us, Gabriel's mother came to sit and rock her child under our ever-watchful eyes. As his breathing and heart rate slowed, she cried tears of both sorrow and joy for this precious child. There wasn't a dry eye in the nursery that night as we continued to care for the rest of our small patients.

Shortly before dawn Gabriel's mother asked me to hold her child. "He's been almost as much your baby as he was mine and I know that you are grieving for him as well," she said. As I sat and rocked Gabriel for the last time I told him goodbye and thanked his mother for allowing me to care for him. As the sun rose on a beautiful summer morning, Gabriel took his last breath and died in his mother's arms.

Over the years I have thought of Gabriel often, wondering what he would have been like had he survived. I also marvel at the fact that this child who had so little, gave so much to so many during his short life. As the sun rises on another beautiful summer morning, I remember that this is the year that Gabriel would have turned twenty-one and I think, *Maybe he really was an angel.*

Mary Stassi, RNC

My Journey Continues

I am six years old. I watch, spellbound, as my grandmother draws up her insulin, wets a piece of cotton, and, after scrubbing a circular patch on her thigh, plunges the needle into her soft flesh.

One day later, *I* wet the cotton and scrub a not-so-perfect circle on Nana's opposite thigh. I watch, with a satisfied smile, as Nana injects herself, right in the middle of my circle.

I am eight years old. My family moves to Butte, into an apartment across from the now-empty hospital where my mom worked as a student nurse. I love to listen to her stories. "We'd take the miners out there for some sunshine," she says, pointing to the second floor windowed solarium.

We walk up the alley. "The kitchen was in there," she says. "Margie and I had to make pudding one day. We took a big taste, and realized that, instead of sugar, we'd put in salt." We laugh, as she points to the place where they dumped the pudding. "Then we had to start all over," she says.

I am eleven years old. We visit our relatives in Columbia Falls. Long after the "lights out" command, my cousin Kathy and I read, by flashlight, under the sheet of our makeshift tent on her twin bed. I read *Cherry Ames: Staff Nurse.*

When we tire of juggling books, flashlight, and sheet, we undo our tent, tuck our books under the bed, and turn out the light. We whisper about what we want to be when we grow up. Kathy wants to be a veterinarian. I want to be a nurse.

I am fourteen years old. In my red and white candy striper pinafore, I feel like I've reached the moon. One year earlier, on my thirteenth birthday, men *did* reach the moon. I stood that day, for what seemed an eternity, beside the television until the exact moment the reporter declared, *"Man on the moon!"* The picture my father snapped memorializes my teenaged indifference: one sock up, one sock down; shoulders slumped; a scowl on my face.

Now, as I pass the hospital sign that says, "No Visitors Under 16," and know that I'm not a visitor but a *volunteer*, I feel like I've achieved the utmost victory.

I am eighteen years old. Quarantined in my dorm room with rubella, three friends put on their new blue and white student nurse uniforms and bring me dinner. On a separate tray, one carries Q-tips, three colors of Jell-O, a can opener and a dollop of mayonnaise.

"This is for the pap smear we're going to do after you eat," Marj says. "And you get to pick your own Jell-O." I laugh along with them, but my focus is on their uniforms. I *can't wait* until I get mine the following year.

I am twenty years old. My patient, eighteen, is in labor with her first child. I've been to the Lamaze classes my mother taught; as students, we served as teaching assistants. But I have never yet witnessed a birth. "Breathe like this," I say, as I gently stroke my patient's legs. Beside her bed, her husband sits in a straight-backed chair, a terrified look on his face.

When the time comes, I accompany my patient into the delivery room, sad that her husband can't join us. Because he hasn't taken childbirth classes, he is denied access. I cup my hand under my patient's neck as she bears down. When her baby's slippery body emerges, I cry.

I am twenty-two years old. My elderly patient lies dying in 302-A, his every breath a struggle. Bleary-eyed after their all-night vigil, his RN daughter and his wife sit beside his bed. Knowing that "home" is across the street, I ask, "Do you want to go home for half-an-hour while I bathe him and change his sheets?" Reluctantly, the wife agrees to accompany her daughter.

I gather linens, and in my haste, realize I've forgotten a washcloth. I hurry down the hall, and when I reenter the room, it's eerily quiet. Walking around the curtain, I see my patient's still body. Tears fill my eyes as I walk to the phone, knowing that, because of me, my patient died alone.

I am twenty-five years old. My heart pounds as I greet the students as they enter the classroom. Tonight I am not an assistant; I am *the* Lamaze teacher. Jan, my supervising instructor, sits quietly beside me as a woman says, "We want to check out this first class before we pay."

"Okay," I reply, feeling my face flush.

After class, the couple stops and pays for the series—an affirmation to me. "I wouldn't have let them do that," Jan says, after the room has emptied. "And next time, don't lecture so much."

Throughout the remaining six weeks, my voice loses its tremulousness. I lecture less. And I thrill at the evaluations I receive at the end of the final class.

I am twenty-nine years old. I am working in a family practice office, and on this particular day, I will be both nurse *and* patient. Undergoing infertility testing, I am scheduled at 1:15 for a post-coital test. All morning I try to convince myself that I can set aside my embarrassment and move from being nurse to patient, and back.

An elderly woman arrives at 1:00 with chest pain. I methodically run her ECG, silently fretting, *This is* my *appointment time.* I worry too much time will pass before my exam.

Forty-five minutes later, my exam is completed. I go back to being a nurse, and prepare the room for the next patient. My stomach quivers as I walk toward our laboratory, anticipating the slide—my cervical mucous and Rich's sperm—that I'm about to see. Turning the corner, I hear Dr. Nevin say, "They're all dead?" to my co-worker Deb. My face blazes.

I am thirty-one years old. Twenty-one of us file upstairs from a basement conference room to the Obstetrics unit. Two weeks ago I made this same trek, as I have so many times before.

Entering labor and delivery, it hits me: *I'm not giving this tour; I'm on this tour.* As we walk into a birthing room, my unborn baby kicks. I look around the room from a brand new perspective.

I am thirty-three years old. No longer a volunteer for the American Red Cross, I am now on staff, and I take two-year-old Eric to his first full day of childcare. I give him a hug and a kiss before he scampers off to play in a home where he's been several times before.

My chest feels tight when I return to the Red Cross office. I've used lancets for finger sticks, but have not used a needle to obtain blood for more than three years. And I haven't used a large, 18-gauge needle, in seven.

I accompany Barb, watching and learning as she moves from donor to donor. When it is my turn, my pulse quickens as I anchor the donor's vein and pierce his skin. Releasing the clamp, I offer a silent prayer of thanks as the warm, red blood fills the tubing and bag.

I am thirty-five years old. Four-year-old Eric and twenty-month-old Colin are asleep as I drive to the hospital in the inky darkness. After a ten-year hiatus from hospital nursing, I am back, working in Obstetrics. There are many changes—new doctors, new chart forms, new medications, and new anesthesia. My first week, I feel overwhelmed and wonder if I can jump in.

After working overtime to complete my paperwork, I visit our OB director. I choke back tears as I say, "Syd's showing me how to stock the labor rooms. I know I need to learn that, but right now, I need to learn how to chart." Jackie agrees, and schedules me extra orientation days.

I am forty-six years old. My patient, hospitalized for preterm labor, and her husband are awake as I creep into their room. Though strangers only hours earlier, we've since shared stories about ourselves and our children in the intimacy that develops from hands on a pregnant belly, and hands arranging linens on a bedside cot.

After adjusting the fetal heart monitor, I ask if they need anything before I turn to leave. "No," they reply. The husband says, "You're the best nurse I've ever met—and I've met a lot."

I am fifty years old. Sharing new life remains magical, but I am tired. I stay on night shift by choice. Each night, driving to work, I silently affirm, *There is energy and healing in my hands.*

I plan that when Colin graduates high school in 2008, I'll earn my get-out-of-nursing-free card. "That'll be thirty years," I say. "Some people get a pension after that long."

I am collecting essays from registered nurses. Reading their stories reminds me of one of my goals for creating this book: inspiring fellow nurses to *stay* in nursing. I know there's life—and nursing—beyond night shift. I decide to stay. And I am glad.

Karen Buley, RN, BSN

We Must Speak Up

"*Who* will answer the call lights?" This question, posed at a 2005 childbirth conference, was the seed for *Nurses on the Run*. Here, nurses share their stories of how they touch our lives from birth to death. They assess us, care for us, comfort and educate us—in clinics, in schools, in hospitals, in prisons, in churches, and in our homes.

It's not surprising that nursing has been voted the "most trusted profession" by Americans in the annual Gallup survey for the seventh consecutive year.[1]

Yet, since 1998, we have been experiencing the longest nursing shortage of the past fifty years. Though once expected to reach a deficit of more than one million nurses by 2016,[2] the economic recession which began in December, 2007 has helped reduce the nursing shortage.[3] In 2007-2008, more than a quarter million RNs entered the hospital workforce. Despite this gain, experts predict a shortage of approximately 260,000 registered nurses by 2025—a magnitude more than twice as large as any nursing shortage experienced since the 1960's.[4]

Our aging population is increasing health care needs; our aging nurses are retiring; job stress, and less than optimal staffing levels and working conditions are creating an exodus of all ages.[5,6] Therefore we must rebuild our nursing workforce, by attracting and educating prospective nurses, and by retaining nurses within their profession.

Attracting people to nursing is not a challenge. In 2008, roughly 100,000 *qualified* applicants were turned away from U.S. associate and baccalaureate degree nursing programs due to lack of space.[7]

Educating future nurses *is* a challenge. Unfilled teaching positions exist, and more are anticipated due to impending teacher retirements. Income disparities make these positions difficult to fill since graduate degree nurses typically earn more in clinical settings than in academia.[8] Budget constraints, lack of training space, and insufficient numbers of hospital training sites add to the problem.[9]

Retaining nurses is also a challenge. A study published in 2002 *Journal of the American Medical Association (JAMA)* reported that, when assigned to more than four patients, for each additional patient, surgical nurses experienced a 15% increase in job dissatisfaction and a 23% increase in burnout.[10] The study also demonstrated that when surgical nurses were assigned more than four patients each, for each additional patient, there was a resulting 7% increased risk of death within thirty days of admission.[11]

A study published in *Health Affairs*, January/February 2006 showed that by increasing RN staffing—where RN levels are low—hospitals could prevent 70,000 complications, 6,700 deaths, and 4.1 million hospital days each year.[12] Though increasing RN staffing would be a monetary investment for hospitals, this study did not examine cost savings associated with decreased nurse turnover, nor did it look at benefits to patients (less absenteeism, decreased pain and suffering) or to hospitals (improved reputation, less liability).[13]

Another study, reported in *Medical Care*, January 2009 suggested that adding 133,000 RNs—to areas of low RN staffing—would save 5,900 lives and decrease hospital days by 3.6 million each year, resulting in an increase of more than $1.5 billion in national productivity.[14] Associated medical savings (before subtracting the cost of additional nurses) are estimated at $6.1 billion. The authors write, "Combining medical savings with increased productivity, these partial estimates of economic value average $57,700 for each of the additional 133,000 RNs."[15] The study did not look at the full economic value of adding RNs, such as cost savings associated with reduced pain and suffering, improved hospital reputation, and reduced nurse turnover.[16]

And nursing turnover is an issue that cannot be ignored. A 2002 article reported replacement costs of recruiting and training RNs at an estimated $42,000 for medical-surgical nurses and $64,000 for specialty nurses.[17]

A July, 2006 survey reported that 55% of surveyed nurses—the majority nurse managers—were planning to retire between 2011 and 2020.[18] In a survey of new nurses published in August, 2009, 37% said they were ready to change jobs.[19] And a January, 2009 *Nursing Economics* article suggests that losing mid-career nurses may be a larger problem than losing new hires.[20]

In a 2009 global study, 92% of more than 2000 nurses from eleven countries said that time constraints keep them from spending time with patients.[21] According to 96%, having more time with patients would have "significant impact" on patients' health.[22]

An American Nurses Association poll conducted between March 31, 2008 and June 5, 2009 found that 52.7% of the 14,993 respondents were currently considering leaving their positions.²³ Inadequate staffing was the reason given by 42.2%.²⁴

What can nurses do?

We can support legislation that mandates safe working conditions for all nurses. We can speak out about safe staffing, and speak in favor of public and private funding for workforce development—for more school nurses, more community nurses, more hospital nurses—and for nursing education.

We can tell the public of the importance of the work we do.²⁵ And we can work together toward eliminating inaccurate portrayals of nursing in the media.²⁶

We can take care of ourselves, both in and out of the workplace. We can work on recognizing and assuming responsibility for our own emotions—and realize that *we,* and not others, control whether we choose to be happy or not.²⁷

There may be days where we run from one patient to the next, without time to stop and chart, without time to stop and eat, and occasionally, with barely a minute to spare to use the restroom, resulting in so-called "nurse's bladder."²⁸ On those days—when we're feeling overwhelmed and overworked—we need to acknowledge the power we have over our own reactions. And move forward with positive energy—one step at a time.

We must take care of both our new nurses *and* our seasoned nurses. If we see a co-worker feeling stressed, we can pitch in and help. By working together, we improve morale, reduce burnout, and provide for better self-care and patient care.²⁹

What can hospitals do?

Hospitals can lengthen residencies for new nurses. Fifty-two hospitals with year-long nurse residencies cited an average nurse turnover of 6% in 2007,[30] significantly less than the 37% who, in *Nursing Outlook* 2009, reported they were ready to change jobs.[31] And a study showed that creating roles for veteran nurses to provide emotional mentorship to new nurses "may go a long way toward improving the retention rates among both groups of nurses."[32]

Hospitals can foster a sense of connection in the workplace.[33] In *Where Have All the Nurses Gone?* Faye Satterly, RN writes, "A happy workforce is the best recruitment tool."[34]

Hospitals can increase RN staffing if needed. When nurses are assigned to larger numbers of patients, there is a resulting increase in job dissatisfaction and burnout.[35] Inadequate staffing was the reason that, in a recent survey, 42.2% of nurses were considering leaving their positions.[36]

Hospitals can improve the ergonomic environment in an effort to retain older nurses;[37] and offer flexible schedules, creative staffing (admission nurse, discharge nurse, nurse educator), and shorter shifts.

What can all of us, as consumers of health care, do?
Become proactive.

Ask hospitals to post their staffing plans—as required by law in certain states.[38] Patronize those hospitals that provide the quality of care you wish to receive. After receiving care, fill out patient questionnaires—give positive feedback and/or constructive suggestions for improvement.

Support legislation that mandates safe working conditions for all nurses. Speak to corporations, foundations, and institutions about the nursing shortage and about creative uses of grant monies—for free or low-cost refresher courses for returning nurses, for hospital residencies for new graduate nurses, or for loan forgiveness programs for graduate degree nurses who become nurse educators.

What is being done?

Monies *are* being invested in nursing education and workplace development by individuals, corporations, foundations, hospitals, colleges and universities.[39,40,41,42] State and federal dollars, including about one hundred million dollars of the economic stimulus plan, have been designated to help alleviate the nursing shortage.[43,44,45,46]

Eight states have enacted legislation to improve ergonomics for nurses.[47] Eleven states have passed safe staffing laws.[48] Fifteen states have enacted legislation regarding mandatory overtime.[49] And at the federal level, more than thirty bills have been introduced in the 2009-2010 Congressional session regarding nursing workforce development, staffing, and nursing education.[50]

Organizations are providing quality care, and earning recognition for their efforts. The American Nurses Credentialing Center (ANCC) awards Magnet® designation to healthcare organizations that demonstrate nursing excellence.[51] Three hundred forty healthcare organizations across the country—and four internationally—have achieved this status.[52]

"*Who* will answer the call lights?" I have worked, and continue to work with many excellent secretaries, surgical techs, nurse techs and LPNs. Yet these stories illustrate how *RNs*—the nucleus of a sound healthcare system—care for us, educate us, comfort and guide us.

We applaud the more than 70% of RNs, who, in a national survey said they would recommend nursing as a viable career choice to a qualified student.[53] We celebrate the strides that have been made on behalf of nurses, but we realize there is more to be done.

"*Together we can change the future, one person at a time,*" writes Pamela F. Cipriano, PhD, RN, FAAN and Editor-in-Chief of *American Nurse Today.*[54]

So we must *all* speak up—and take action. Together, we must work to ensure that when the situation or setting dictates, an *RN* will be there to attend to us in our time of need.*

*See page 139 for endnotes

Permissions

An APRN's Journey. © 2007. Anne Scott Fredrickson.

The Best Part. © 2007. Adrienne Muhammad.

A Call to Pastoral Nursing. © 2008. Michaelle Washington.

From the Beginning. © 2008. Shirley Oscarson Wood.

I Pass on the Torch. © 2008. Marguerite Oberle Thomas.

More than Making Beds and Emptying Bedpans. © 2009. Drew Payne.

My Cosmic Uncle Sam. © 2008. Liza Leukhardt.

My Heart Sings. © 2009. Victoria Powell.

My Journey Continues. © 2007. Karen Buley.

Nora. © 2008. Marjorie Rothermel.

The Notebook. © 2009. Joanne Cherry.

The Nurse's High. © 2008. Lucy May J. Colegado.

A Nurse's Journey: Expectations, Hope, and Compromise. © 2008. Keith Carlson.

Nurses in Bald Places. Reprinted with permission of *Portland*, University of Portland, Portland, OR. © 2007. Hob Osterlund.

Nursing in the Big House. © 2006. Sara Stassen.

Nursing is about the Contribution You Make...Whether You Know It or Not. © 2009. Stephanie A. Lopuszynski.

Of buck teeth, nebulizers, and the Tooth Fairy. Reprinted with permission of *NEA Today*, NEA, Washington, DC. © 2008. Maggie Compton Beall.

An Old Soldier Heads Home. © 2007. William Robert Moore.

Contributors

Maggie Compton Beall, BS, MA, RN,BC is a certified school nurse practitioner. She is a part-time faculty member of Drexel University, and previously served on the faculties of West Virginia University and the University of Pittsburgh. She serves as the President of the Department of Pupil Services of the Pennsylvania State Education Association, and is the liaison from the National Association of School Nurses to the National Education Association Board of Directors. Maggie was named "Pennsylvania School Nurse of the Year" in 1998-1999, and in 2004 she received the PSEA Nurse Leadership Excellence Award. Maggie has three children, Jonathan, Gretchen and husband Moritz, and Star. She adores grandson, Max, "sunshine boy!"

Keith Carlson, RN, BSN is a nurse, writer, blogger and entrepreneur. His work has been included in nursing anthologies published by Kaplan Publishing, and he was the recipient of the first Nurse Blogger Scholarship awarded by Value Care Value Nurses, the nursing arm of the Service Employees International Union. Please feel free to visit his blog at http://digitaldoorway. blogspot.com and his personal website at http:// keithcarlson.vpweb.com. Keith can be reached at nursekeith@gmail.com.

Joanne Cherry, RN, BA, QTTP (Qualified Therapeutic Touch Practitioner) started her nursing career as an LPN in Cleveland, Ohio in 1963. She moved to Florida in 1969, and became an RN in 1978. As a hospital nurse, Joanne worked in a variety of areas, from neonatal intensive care to geriatrics. After having children, Joanne switched to Home Health Care, which allowed her more flexibility with scheduling and child care. For the past eight years, Joanne has worked for Suncoast Hospice, and though she considered retiring last year, she instead scaled back to a two-day work week. Working every Saturday and Sunday gives her the opportunity to pursue her hobbies during the week—reading, writing, and gardening. Joanne continues to be surprised by what she learns from her patients, and by what they tell her that nurses really give to them. Joanne can be reached at jcgypsy102@aol.com.

Lucy May J. Colegado, RN, BSN earned her BSN from Adventist University of the Philippines in 1993. She has been a bedside nurse for more than ten years. The first four years of her career were spent working in a private hospital in Pasay City, Philippines—in labor and delivery, pediatrics, and ICU. She has been working in a Southern California medical center for the past six years, the first few months in a medical surgical ICU, and now in a medical intermediate telemetry unit.

Christine Contillo, RN-BC, BS, BSN is a certified Community Health Nurse. She received a BS from Cornell University, and earned her BSN from The Catholic University of America in 1979. Prior to her current position in Columbia University Student Health Services, Chris worked Labor and Delivery; was a parent-educator; and a Public Health Nurse Supervisor in Paramus, New Jersey. Chris likes to hike, knit and write, and she and her husband recently adopted a dog that had been abandoned in Beirut, Lebanon. They have three grown children. Christine can be reached at NurseMomNJ@aol.com.

Karen M. Cooper, RN, BSN, MA has a Master's Degree in Holistic Health Education and has had an eclectic nursing career. Her experiences include Neonatal Intensive Care, Infant Development, Women and Newborn care, Medical Sales, Cancer Survivorship, Pediatric Hospice, and she has served as Breast Care Coordinator at the University of

Wisconsin Hospital and Clinics in Madison. Karen advocates Primary Care Nursing, Integrative Medicine, and teaches Mindful Yoga. She has a private Integrative Health practice in Madison, Izumi Joi, which emphasizes working with companies to improve the health of their employees through worksite wellness programs, and with individual clients who wish to restore their power and experience the joy of better health. Karen can be reached at mindful-nurse@gmail.com.

Anne Scott Fredrickson, MSN, APRN,BC is a graduate of Florida State University in Tallahassee, Florida and George Mason University in Fairfax, Virginia. She is a Psychiatric Clinical Nurse Specialist in Adult Psychiatric and Mental Health Nursing. After retiring from INOVA Alexandria Hospital she continues to maintain a small private mental health practice in Springfield, Virginia. She was a Magnet Recognition Award Appraiser from 1993 until the end of 2006. Anne can be reached at annescottf@verizon.net.

Amy Nelson Knutson, RN, BSN is a school nurse, mom, actress and creator of artful objects. After enjoying worldly adventures as a young nurse, she is thrilled to be back near extended family in her hometown of Polson, Montana where she lives with her husband. Both children are off on their own adventures now, seeking their versions of the fulfillment that Amy has enjoyed throughout her college years and nursing career. Having collected people and stories all her life, Amy says some of her most treasured collectibles are the patients who piqued her memory banks while sharing themselves and the emotions encircling their lives. Her work as a school nurse keeps her laughing, loving the diversity that the nursing profession affords, and contemplating penning further reflections of her diverse career. Amy can be reached at knuthaus@polson.net.

Liza Leukhardt, MS, RN, CHPN continues to work as a homecare and hospice nurse at VNA Healthcare in Waterbury, Connecticut. She is a counselor for Camp Jonathan—a camp for bereaved children, is certified to teach chair yoga to challenged populations, and she volunteers as a literacy counselor for at-risk youth. She is pursuing a degree as doctor of naturopathy, and recently began work on a master's degree in grief counseling. She will be working toward certification in reflexology this fall, and hopes to become certified as a holistic health nurse in the near future. Liza can be reached at lleukhardt@gmail.com.

Stephanie A. Lopuszynski, RN, BSN, BS earned a degree in Journalism from Bowling Green State University in the 1980's. Her business career began in textiles—in training and management development—but led to a position with a world-renowned consulting firm focused on quality improvement processes. While volunteering for a local hospice in the 1990's, Stephanie discovered a love for patient care, and everything changed. She earned her BSN at Kennesaw State University, and began her nursing career at St. Joseph's Hospital in Atlanta. There, she held positions as a Patient Care Technician, Night Shift Charge Nurse and Care Coordinator with cancer and medical-surgical patients, and Float Pool RN, before becoming the first full-time Admission Nurse. During her time in that role, she helped initiate the hospital's minimal lift program, which uses specialized devices and training to ensure safety for caregivers while mobilizing patients. In 2007, Stephanie conducted a Robert Wood Johnson Foundation research study titled "Wisdom at Work: Retaining Experienced Nurses at the Bedside." A nurse for thirteen years, she now works as a Clinical Consultant for Diligent Services. Stephanie can be reached at stephski@mindspring.com.

William Robert Moore, RN, SFO works at the Minnesota Veterans Home in Minneapolis. He and his wife are members of the Mary, Queen of Peace Fraternity of the Secular Franciscan Order. Secular Franciscans are lay people who together strive to live out charity; they make a Profession to observe the gospel by following the example of Saint Francis of Assisi who made Christ the inspiration and center of his life. Will has authored many articles for their Fraternity newsletter; is an active contributor to The Secular Franciscan Order Queen of Peace Region email Forum; and enjoys reading, writing, running, and bridge. He and Eileen have three children. Will can be reached at wemoore@usfamily.net.

Adrienne Muhammad, RN, MSN, Women's Health NP, APNP was born in Chicago to working class parents. She worked as a labor and delivery nurse for ten years before moving to Madison, Wisconsin to go to graduate school. Currently, she works as a women's health nurse practitioner in college health. She enjoys reading literary fiction, writing, traveling, watching indie films, and listening to R &B oldies and world music.

Hob Osterlund, APRN,C is a clinical nurse specialist in pain and palliative care at the Queen's Medical Center in Honolulu. Since 1998, she's been performing a popular one-woman comedy for audiences all over North America featuring her alter ego "Ivy Push, RN." She's the Principal Investigator in the COMIC (comedy in chemotherapy) Study, a randomized trial looking at the impact of comedy on the symptoms of cancer and chemotherapy. Hob is also the founder, president and producer for the "Chuckle Channel" (www.chucklechannel.com) closed-circuit comedy programming for hospitals all over the country. Hob can be reached at chucklechannel@hawaii.rr.com.

Drew Payne, RGN, EMB 219, EMB 998, BSc (Hons) has worked in HIV, Orthopaedics, Tissue Viability, and Trauma care. In the community he has worked as a Primary Care Nurse, Telephone Triage Nurse, GP Out-of-Hours Service and locum nurse for a Walk-In Centre. In addition to his Registered General Nurse (RGN) qualification, Drew holds specialist qualifications in Orthopaedic Nursing, Teaching and Assessing, and a BSc in Health. He is a regular contributor to *Nursing Times*, *Nursing Standard*, and *FS Magazine*—a national men's health magazine. For the *Nursing Standard* he has three times been a guest editor. At present, he works as an Audit Nurse and Trainer. Drew can be reached at drew.london@gmail.com.

Victoria Powell, RN, CCM, LNCC, CNLCP, MSCC, CEAS[II] is the President of VP Medical Consulting (www.VP-Medical.com), a nurse consulting firm in Central Arkansas. She and her team of nurses provide services to employers, insurance companies, attorneys and the general public such as case management and life care planning. Patient advocacy is the mainstay of the business. When she is not providing advocacy services to her patients, Victoria can often be found speaking on nurse consulting related topics, playing with her grandchildren or traveling the world with her husband. Victoria can be reached at victoria@vp-medical.com.

Marjorie Rothermel, RN, BA graduated from Presbyterian-St. Luke's Hospital School of Nursing in Chicago,

Illinois in 1962. She married in 1961 and raised five boys. Through the years, she worked in med-surg, a nursing home, and home health. In 1969 she and her family moved to Montana, and in 1986 Marje earned a BA in social work and English writing from Carroll College in Helena. For several years she worked as a journalist for a newspaper and various magazines. In 2000 she received certification in parish nursing and has served as parish nurse for a small church in Missoula ever since. Marje can be reached at marjroth@centric.net.

Sara Stassen RN, BSN graduated from the University of Virginia's Second Degree Nursing program in May 2004. Following graduation, she worked for three years in the infirmary in a maximum security prison. After relocating to Houston, Texas she re-entered the hospital setting at Memorial Hermann's Epilepsy Monitoring Center where she works with a pediatric as well as an adult population. Sara can be reached at sestassen@yahoo.com.

Mary E. Stassi, RNC is a Nursing Educator, author and professional speaker. She lives at Twelve Oaks Farm, outside of Saint Louis, Missouri with her husband, daughter and a small herd of horses. Most weekends, she keeps busy traveling to horse shows. Mary can be reached at mstassi@stchas.edu.

Marguerite Oberle Thomas, RN, BScN is a graduate of Georgian College, Humber College and Ryerson University. She worked as a Public Health Nurse for twenty-one years, specializing in the Prevention of Falls in Older Adults at the Grey Bruce Health Unit from 2001-

2008. During 2004-2005, Thomas was Program Coordinator for the "Stay on Your Feet" Falls Prevention in Older
Adults rural demonstration project. Thomas, now retired
and acting as a consultant, has dedicated time for publi-
cations and presentations on a variety of health and nursing related topics. She is a strong advocate for The Truth
About Nursing: www.truthaboutnursing.org. Marguerite
can be reached at marguerite@thomas.name.

Barbara H. Toenyes, RN, BSN has worked in many areas
of nursing throughout her forty-one-year career. Her
passions are family, decorating her home, reading,
current events, and volunteering with the American Red
Cross. When she isn't working, she likes to take advan-
tage of the Montana outdoors—birding, hiking and
canoeing. She and her husband, John, are looking forward to retiring and traveling.

Helen N. Turner, DNP, RN-BC, PCNS-BC is the Pediatric
Pain Management Clinical Nurse Specialist at Doern-
becher Children's Hospital/OHSU. She is responsible
for managing pain care for children during their hospital stay as well as coordinating care for children with
chronic pain who are seen in the Pediatric Pain
Clinic. Helen received her BSN from Montana State University in 1980, her MSN from the University of California, San Francisco in 1990, and her DNP from Oregon
Health & Science University in 2009. She lectures
extensively on pediatric pain management. Helen can be
reached at mtgrl2000@yahoo.com.

Michaelle Washington, RN, MSN is the Pastoral Nurse
for Unity Church of Chatsworth, California. Previously

she served as Parish Nurse for Unity Christian Church of Battle Creek and on the Parish Nurse team at Christ Church Unity in Kansas City, Missouri, where she and her husband were the voices of "Good News PLUS" on Gospel Radio KPRT 1590 AM. Prior to nursing, Michaelle's background included corporate management and human resources. She is a member of The American Holistic Nursing Association, The Association of Applied Therapeutic Humor, the World Laughter Tour, and is the author of *A Joy Filled Tool Box*~a guide for using the tools of breath, laughter, belief and positive attitude to live a happier, more productive life. Michaelle can be reached at nursingspirit@yahoo.com.

Joanne Whary, MSN, FNP-BC has depended on God and her Christian values as the cornerstones of her life. Of German descent, she was born and raised in southeastern Pennsylvania, in a residential area that resembled the Levittowns of the era. She graduated from the Reading Hospital School of Nursing in 1969, and in 1997 she earned a Bachelor's Degree of Nursing from Millersville University. Five years later, she earned her Master's Degree from Widener University. This year marks the forty-year milestone of her nursing career. Joanne and her husband—who will celebrate their fortieth wedding anniversary in 2010—have one son, one daughter, and four grandchildren. Joanne is an avid reader, loves to cook, and enjoys walking, bicycling, and traveling. She has visited Europe, the Caribbean, Hawaii, and the South Pacific. Though looking forward to retirement, she still has the desire to continue her career for another ten years. She believes that she can still make a difference, and her future goals include mission work and volunteerism. Joanne can be reached at jwhary@paonline.com.

Shirley Oscarson Wood, MNEd, CNS, RN graduated from Montana State University in 1962. She lives in Middle-field, Ohio and is a retired maternal/child nurse, a published author, and a Professor Emeriti at Kent State University. An active volunteer throughout her nursing career, Shirley continues to serve on the Amish Birth Center Medical board and on the board of the Ohio Chapter of the March of Dimes. Raised on a wheat farm and cattle ranch in Malta, Montana, she enjoys reading, traveling, and spending time with her granddaughters. Shirley can be reached at shirleyshirleyo@aol.com.

About the Editor

Karen Buley, RN, BSN graduated from Montana State University in 1978. She has worked in hospitals, in a physicians' office, for the American Red Cross, and she taught Lamaze classes for sixteen years. Karen continues to care for new families and their babies in Missoula, Montana.

Her publishing credits include *American Nurse Today*, *A Cup of Comfort for Nurses*, *Directions in Nursing*, *Family Circle*, *Holiday Voices*, the *Missoulian*, *Montana Voices*, and *Story Circle Journal*.

Karen credits her roots to Butte, America, birthplace of her parents and her home throughout most of her childhood. She enjoys reading, writing, hiking, and volunteer work. Having lived in Missoula—home of the University of Montana Grizzlies—for the past thirty-one years, Karen cheers for the home team. *However*, when the Grizzlies play the Montana State Bobcats—her alma mater—she proudly wears her blue and gold and roots for the Cats. In summer, 2009 she resurrected her cleats to play co-rec soccer with her husband, Rich, and their sons, Eric and Colin. Eric is a student at Pacific Lutheran University in Tacoma, Washington; Colin is a student at Seattle University. Karen lives by her motto, "You can't win if you don't try." She can be reached at kmb@karenbuley.com.

Endnotes

[1] Saad, L. Nurses Shine, Bankers Slump in Ethics Ratings. November 24, 2008. http://www.gallup.com/poll/ 112264/ Nurses-Shine-While-Bankers-Slump-Ethics-Ratings.aspx. Accessed December 15, 2008.

[2] Dohm, A., Shniper, L. Occupational Employment Projections to 2016. *Monthly Labor Review*. 2007; 130:86-125.

[3] Buerhaus, P., Auerbach, D., Staiger, D. The Recent Surge in Nurse Employment: Causes and Implications. *Health Affairs-Web Exclusive*. June 12, 2009. 28:w657-w668.

[4] Buerhaus, P. ibid. pw663-w664.

[5] Pellico, L., Brewer, C., Kovner, C. What newly licensed registered nurses have to say about their first experiences. *Nursing Outlook*. 2009; 57:194-203.

[6] Coshow, S., Davis, P., Wolosin, R. The 'Big Dip': Decrements in RN Satisfaction at Mid-Career. *Nursing Economics*. 2009; 27:15-18.

[7] Carlson, J. Group Pushes Nurse Shortage as Key Issue. February 23, 2009.
http://www.modernhealthcare.com/apps/pbcs.dll/ article?AID=/20090223/REG/302239958. Accessed February 24, 2009.

[8] American Association of Colleges of Nursing (AACN). Nursing Faculty Shortage. Updated June 2009. http://www.aacn.nche.edu/Media/FactSheets/ FacultyShortage.htm. Accessed August 19, 2009.

[9] American Association of Colleges of Nursing (AACN). ibid.

[10] Aiken, L., Clarke, S., Sloane, D., Sochalski, J., Silber, J. Hospital Nurse Staffing and Patient Mortality, Nurse Burnout, and Job Dissatisfaction. *Journal of the American Medical Association (JAMA)*. 2002; 288:1987-1993.

[11] Aiken, L. ibid. p1991.

[12] Needleman, J., Buerhaus, P., Stewart, M., Zelevinsky, K., Mattke, S. Nurse Staffing in Hospitals: Is There a Business Case for Quality? *Health Affairs*. 2006; 25:204-211.

[13] Needleman, J. ibid. p209-210.

[14] Dall, T., Chen, Y., Seifert, R., Maddox, P., Hogan, P. The Economic Value of Professional Nursing. *Medical Care*. 2009; 47:97-104.

[15] Dall, T. ibid. p101.

[16] Dall, T. ibid. p103.

[17] Aiken, L. op.cit. p1992.

[18] American Association of Colleges of Nursing (AACN). Nursing Shortage. Updated June 2009. http://www.aacn.nche.edu/Media/FactSheets/Nursing Shortage.htm. Accessed August 19, 2009.

[19] Pellico, L. op cit. p200.

[20] Coshow, S. op. cit. p15.

[21] International Council of Nurses (ICN). Nurses in the Workplace: Expectations and Needs. 2009. http://www.icn.ch/ Workplace_survey2009.htm. Accessed August 22, 2009.

[22] International Council of Nurses (ICN). ibid.

[23] American Nurses Association (ANA). Safe Nursing Staffing Poll Results. 2009. http://www.safestaffingsaveslives.org/WhatisANA Doing/PollResults.aspx. Accessed August 22, 2009.

[24] American Nurses Association (ANA). ibid.

[25] Buresh, B., Gordon, S. *From Silence to Voice: What Nurses Know and Must Communicate to the Public*. Ithaca, NY: Cornell University Press, 2000.

[26] Summers, S., Summers, H. *Saving Lives: Why the Media's Portrayal of Nurses Puts Us All at Risk*. New York: Kaplan Publishing, 2009.

[27] Scott, E. Get smart: Increase your emotional intelligence. *American Nurse Today*. 2009; 4:14-15.

28 Fitzgerald, S. Bladder Health: How to avoid 'nurse's bladder' with basic self-maintenance. *American Journal of Nursing.* 2005; 105:104.

29 Scott, E. op. cit. p14.

30 Madkour, R. Nursing shortage: 1 in 5 quits within first year, study shows. *USA Today.* February 15, 2009. http:// www.usatoday.com/news/health/2009-02-15-nursing-shortage_N.htm?POE+click-refer. Accessed February 18, 2009.

31 Pellico, L. op. cit. p200.

32 Erickson, R., Grove, W. Why Emotions Matter: Age, Agitation, and Burnout Among Registered Nurses. *OJIN: The Online Journal of Issues in Nursing.* October 29, 2007. http://www.nursingworld.org/MainMenuCategories/ ANAMarketplace/ANAPeriodicals/OJIN/TableofContents/ vol132008/No1Jan08/ArticlePreviousTopic/Why EmotionsMatterAgeAgitationandBurnoutAmong RegisteredNurses.aspx. Accessed January 28, 2008.

33 Manion, J., Bartholomew, K. Community in the Workplace: A Proven Retention Strategy. *The Journal of Nursing Administration (JONA).* 2004; 34:46-53.

34 Satterly, F. *Where Have All the Nurses Gone? The Impact of the Nursing Shortage on American Healthcare.* Amherst, New York: Prometheus Books, 2004.

35 Improving the Quality of Care for Millions of Americans. *American Nurses Association.* June 2008. http://www.safestaffingsaveslives.org/Documents/ SSBrochure.aspx. Accessed October 8, 2008.

36 American Nurses Association (ANA). Safe Nursing Staffing Poll Results. op. cit.

37 Buerhaus, P. op. cit. pw664-w665.

38 Haebler, J. Safe Nurse Staffing Continues... *Capitol Update.* 2009. http://www.rnaction.org/site/ PageServer? pagename=CUP_07_09_IntheStates_ SafeNursingStaffin. Accessed August 22, 2009.

[39] Rojas, R. Preventive Medicine for A Shortage Of Nurses. *Washington Post*. July 23, 2009. http://www. washingtonpost.com/wpdyn/content/article/2009/07/ 21/AR2009072103740.html. Accessed July 23, 2009.

[40] Regional Foundations Collaborate in National Effort to Build Nursing Workforce Capacity. *Robert Wood Johnson Foundation Newsroom*. August 20, 2009. http://www.rwjf. org/pr/product.jsp?id=47548. Accessed August 22, 2009.

[41] Pope, J. Grant may help trim Louisiana nursing shortage. *Times-Picayune*. January 29, 2008. http://www. nola.com/timespic/stories/index.ssf?/base/news26/ 1201587653241850.xml&coll=1. Accessed February 5, 2008.

[42] Alexander, L. Nurses Believe Public Has Positive Image of Nursing, Thanks to Johnson & Johnson Nursing Campaign. *Nursing Economics*. August 2, 2005. http://www. nursingeconomics.net/cgibin/WebObjects/NECJournal. woa/wa/viewSection?tName=newsArticle&od_id=805314 846&s_id=1073744453. Accessed September 3, 2009.

[43] Beltran, J. Iowa and Nation Face Severe Nursing Shortage. February 22, 2008. http://biz.yahoo.com/ap/080222/ ia_nursing_shortage.html?.v=1. Accessed February 26, 2008.

[44] http://www.nursing.illinois.gov. Accessed September 3, 2009.

[45] State, Health Officials Address Severe Nursing Shortage. *Southern Maryland Online*. February 7, 2008. http:// somd. com/news/headlines/2008/7158.shtml. Accessed February 26, 2008.

[46] Dunham, W. US healthcare system pinched by nursing shortage. *Reuters*. March 9, 2009. http://www. reuters.com/article/ healthNews/ idUSTRE5270VC20090309. Accessed March 16, 2009.

[47] Conant, R. ANA Supports Safe Patient Handling Measures in Congress To Improve Safety of Nurses and Patients. *Capitol Update.* 2009. http://www.rnaction.org/site/PageServer?pagename=CUP_07_09_LegUpdate_ANA SupportSafePatientHandling. Accessed August 22, 2009.

[48] Haebler, J. op. cit.

[49] Sixel, L. No more mandatory overtime for nurses. *Houston Chronicle.* September 2, 2009. http://www.chron.com/disp/ story.mpl/business/sixel/6600043.html. Accessed September 3, 2009.

[50] Advanced Bill Summary & Status Search for the 111th Congress (2009-2010). *The Library of Congress Thomas.* 2009. http://thomas.loc.gov. Accessed August 28, 2009.

[51] American Nurses Credentialing Center (ANCC). 2009. http://www.nursecredentialing.org/Magnet/FindaMagnetFacility.aspx. Accessed August 17, 2009.

[52] American Nurses Credentialing Center (ANCC). ibid.

[53] Buerhaus, P., Donelan, K., Ulrich, B., Norman, L., Dittus, R. State of the Registered Nurse Workforce in the United States. *Nursing Economics.* 2006; 24:6-12.

[54] Cipriano, P. Retaining our talent. *American Nurse Today.* 2006; 1:10.

CPSIA information can be obtained at www.ICGtesting.com
Printed in the USA
238380LV00002B/2/P